The Power of Dopamine

Scientifically-Proven Techniques to Boost Mood, Increase Motivation, and (Finally) Finding Balance in a Distracted World, without Negative Habits

Logan Mind

A Gift for You!

Emotional Intelligence for Social Success

Here's what you'll find in the book:

• Unlock the keys to **understanding** your emotions and using them to **connect** with others.

• Discover **strategies** for building stronger relationships, both personally and professionally.

• Learn how to **navigate** social situations with greater ease and confidence.

Just click or follow the below link to start your journey to social **success**:

https://pxl.to/loganmindfreebook

Download your 3 FREE EXTRAS too!

These valuable extras are designed to complement the **insights** from the book and provide practical tools for implementing what you learn. Together, they form a comprehensive **guide** to building and sustaining emotional intelligence over time.

The extras are:

• A downloadable and practical PDF 21-Day Challenge for the book

• The text "101+ Micro-Habits for Sustaining Long-Term Dopamine Balance"

• Quick Habit Checklist for Consistent Dopamine Levels

Just click or follow the below link to gain instant **access** to the extras:

https://pxl.to/12-tpod-lm-extras

Other Books

Thank you for choosing this **book** as part of your life-learning **journey**. If you're interested in continuing to strengthen your **mind**, my other books may offer you just what you're looking for. With the Calm Your Mind NOW! series, you can learn how to **master** emotions through "Letting Go" or reshape your thoughts through "Rewire Your Brain." If overcoming everyday **fears** is your focus, "Overcoming Social Anxiety" provides actionable insights to help build your **confidence**.

For those deeply invested in self-improvement and healing emotional wounds, the Heal Your Mind NOW series, particularly "How to Heal from Family Trauma," will guide you through the steps to mending personal struggles rooted in your past. And if you seek a **boost** to your daily self-worth, the Improve Yourself NOW series, specifically "You Are Amazing," is a great start.

Ready to discover more? Simply:

• Follow the provided link.

• Click on "All My Books."

• Select titles that speak to you.

• Find my contact information at the end of the linked page.

Check out all my books and contacts here:

https://pxl.to/LoganMind

Help Me!

When you're done reading, if **you're satisfied** with this book, I kindly ask for just a few moments of your time. Your feedback, no matter how brief, can make a world of difference.

Why?

• You're supporting a dream, and helping an independent author like myself continue creating work that speaks to you and other readers like you.

• **Your voice** has a significant impact, **sharing** it **helps** future readers discover this story.

If you have suggestions for improvement or other thoughts to share, remember that your insights **are incredibly valuable**—please feel free to reach out using the contact details you'll find at the link below. I want to continue growing, learning, and creating for you.

It only takes a second and **truly means the world** to me.

Visit this link to leave feedback:

https://pxl.to/12-tpod-lm-review

Join my Review Team!

A huge **thank** you for picking up my book! Your **interest** and support mean the world. I'd love to **invite** you to join my Review Team. If you're someone who loves to **dive** into new stories and share your thoughts, this team is perfect for you. Plus, it comes with a perk — you'll get a **free** copy of my upcoming book in exchange for an honest review. Your **feedback** is invaluable and helps me **improve** with each new release.

It's simple to join:

• Click the link below.

• Sign up to ensure you receive notifications when a new book is ready.

• Look out for a special email from me with details on accessing your free copy.

Enjoy the read and thank you in advance for your reviews!

Check out the team at this link:

https://pxl.to/loganmindteam

Introduction

Imagine waking up every morning dragging your feet, feeling no **excitement** for the day ahead. Ever wonder why some days you're overflowing with **motivation** while others feel like you're trudging through mud? Yeah, I've been there too. I think that's why you're here—because honestly, who wouldn't want to grab hold of a little more motivation? And sure, there's no magic wand, but there is science—good ol' dependable science—that might just be the key to figuring it all out.

So, what's this all about? It's about **dopamine**. You know, that chemical everyone keeps talking about. It's like that behind-the-scenes director making sure you feel rewarded or, just as often, making sure you crave something more. This book? All about exploring how dopamine truly works in our lives—and, more importantly, how you can make it serve you better instead of letting it push you around.

Before we dive deeper, I've spent years surrounded by thoughts, debates, and late-night conversations all circling one central question: Why do we do the things we do? From being knee-deep in psychology books to debating philosophy over endless cups of coffee, I've realized something simple and powerful—most of what drives us can be tied back to those biochemical processes that happen right in our brain. Sounds pretty heavy, huh? But let me put it as simply as possible: When you better understand dopamine, you stand a better chance at steering your life in the direction you want.

But where's the catch? Well, it's our modern world, isn't it? Endless pinging from phones, quick fixes at every corner, an almost-always-on culture—doesn't it feel a bit like running a never-ending race?

And you know who's pulling the strings most of the time? Dopamine. It's behind those "gotta check my phone again" moments and the "just one more episode" marathons. It keeps you stuck chasing mini-pleasures, often at the expense of deeper, longer-lasting satisfaction. What I want to do in this book is get into the nitty-gritty of how all that stimulus affects your brain, makes you chase quick highs, and then leaves you wanting more. And—I won't lie—it messes with your balance. It creates such sensitivity in your reward systems that before you know it, you're overloading, and in some cases, burning out completely.

So, how do you fight that? Well, by rethinking some habits, understanding what's happening under the hood, and then figuring out how to put that knowledge to work for you. But it isn't all bad news—it's not like I'm about to pitch some outlandish idea where you have to live off the grid or avoid television altogether. It's really about **balance**, about catching yourself right before you tip over the edge, and learning to play by your rules—not just obeying some chemical dictator in your head.

That brings us to our main challenge: balancing that powerful effect dopamine has on you. If for a moment it sounds impossible to fend off all the **distractions**, consider this—what if you could just tweak things a little? What if understanding how attention and motivation works could explain why some days you feel unstoppable and others like you're sinking? Could be that with just the right insights, you'd build healthier **routines** and find out just how motivated you can really be, naturally, without needing that extra coffee or some other crutch.

But, okay, I get where you might be coming from. "I've tried everything before, and nothing sticks," you might be thinking. Don't get me wrong—everyone's approach to improving themselves is different, but some strategies out there feel, well, scripted. They sell you fluffy ideas that might work great in theory but not in real life. What's frustrating—truly frustrating—is when all those promises of quick fixes fall flat, leaving you right back where you started. If that's been your experience, I totally get it. If you're skeptical, it's because too often those so-called solutions ignore the brain's delicate chemistry—the same chemistry we're tackling here. We aren't pushing band-aids or magic pills in this book. This is about gathering what works, why it works, and mixing in the **science** in a way you can use tomorrow, the next day, or even right now.

So, here's the thing. This book isn't just me sharing theories from some ivory tower or parroting things I've read. I've seen these principles play out in real life too many times to count. From executive coaching to personal mentoring, I've walked alongside folks who figured out not just what dopamine was doing with their moods and decisions, but how to make that knowledge matter, to make it count where it matters most—every day of their lives. It's an amazing feeling, to put into place what you thought was only brain chemistry talk, only to see it change your life. This can become your guide, your map, not someone else's overly polished version. It's all quite doable once you understand—and believe in—the process.

I won't lie—this will take some thinking, a bit of introspection, and yes, a willing mind to maybe approach things a little differently. But if you keep with me, if together we take a look at this peculiar molecule that's influencing you, then you'll likely find that the roots of **motivation**, mood, and balance—well, they aren't as elusive as they once seemed.

So here we are—welcome to your ground zero of understanding just how much this tiny chemical shapes your life. I think of it as learning to hack your own brain, in the best possible way. And you're not doing it alone—I'll be right here with you.

Chapter 1: Understanding Dopamine

Ever wondered what truly **drives** you to chase after a goal or makes you feel on top of the world when you **achieve** something? Here's a hint—it's that little spark in your brain called **dopamine**. I've always been fascinated by how this tiny chemical seems to pull so many strings behind the scenes. But it goes way beyond just making you happy. It **shapes** how you think, what **motivates** you, and even those snap decisions you didn't think twice about.

You're about to get a ringside seat to why you often find yourself doing what you do. This chapter will open your eyes to how dopamine functions like a hidden **control** center, guiding your moods, your **actions**, and the **rewards** you chase. Ready to get to know your brain just a bit better? I promise it's worth the time.

The Function of Dopamine in the Brain

Alright, so **dopamine**. You've probably heard the name tossed around a lot, especially when talking about mood and pleasure. But what exactly does this chemical do? Well, at its core, dopamine is like a messenger that zips around your brain delivering "feel good" signals. Let's dive into how it actually works.

Dopamine plays a starring role in your brain's **reward system**. Picture this: you're faced with a choice between two tasks—one's fun, the other, not so much. The anticipation of doing the fun one? That's dopamine chatting away. When you **accomplish** something important or take a bite of delicious food—bam! A little burst of dopamine gets released in your noggin. It's why a good meal or crossing something off your to-do list feels so darn satisfying. Dopamine sends signals that tell you, "Hey, you did something awesome. Let's do more of this."

In a way, dopamine is your brain's own personal cheerleader, giving you a mental high five whenever you do something positive, egging you on to repeat behaviors that keep you happy and thriving. Reward-driven activities aren't just physical; even social interactions or learning can trigger this dopamine reward mechanism. Think of it as a pat on the back from your brain every time something enjoyable or beneficial happens in your life.

Now, how exactly does this info zip around? That's where dopamine's role in **communication** comes into play.

Dopamine doesn't fly solo in your brain. It's more like a messenger traveling between neurons to share crucial info. These neurons, or brain cells, chat with each other by passing around chemicals—in this case, dopamine. You've got specific neurons in different parts of the brain that release and receive dopamine. When dopamine floats from one neuron to the next, it's like passing notes via paper airplanes between two buddies in class—it keeps your brain in sync.

This nifty little system influences a ton of what you do day-to-day. Feeling **motivated** to go for a run, feeling satisfied with the project you just wrapped up, or being able to guess a friend's next move during a conversation—all these actions rely on dopamine acting as this go-between for your brain cells. It ties your actions to the dopamine release, building an association like, "Oh, this felt good last time, maybe I should do it again." It also shapes habits over time, which can both help and hurt you, depending on the behavior encouraged by that dopamine release.

Just when you were getting the hang of how dopamine lets neurons chat, this chemical also has a job at particular spots in the brain. These areas are central hubs where dopamine gets cooked up and put to use.

Different parts of your brain crank out dopamine and use it for various tasks. One key area is the ventral tegmental area—or VTA for short. Think of VTA like a dopamine factory; it's the part of your brain that pumps out dopamine when your brain thinks there's a **reward** coming your way. This place is especially active when you're craving something, say a slice of pizza, or when you're super pumped about an upcoming event.

Then there's the nucleus accumbens, sort of like the storehouse where dopamine takes action. It's particularly key to processing all that pleasure and reward stuff, making sure the feel-good vibes actually happen. And don't forget the prefrontal cortex—this one links up the dopamine system to **decision-making**, helping figure out what you'll do to reach a goal, rewarding you for solving problems, and honing in on focus.

So, thanks to all these areas—the VTA, nucleus accumbens, and prefrontal cortex—dopamine ties together your desires, decisions, and **habits**. In other words, dopamine's pretty much pulling the strings behind a lot of what you think, do, and feel. Pretty cool, right?

How Dopamine Influences Mood and Motivation

Ever wonder why some days you just feel great for no reason, while other days, it seems like nothing can cheer you up? A lot of that has to do with **dopamine**, the brain's own way of influencing your emotions. Basically, whenever you experience something enjoyable—whether it's savoring a hot cup of coffee or laughing at that one joke your friend always tells—dopamine's the chemical that fires up in your brain. It's like getting a little **mood** boost every time, making those moments feel a lot better.

But here's the catch. When dopamine's out of whack, either too high or too low, things go a bit sideways. You know those days where you're just flat-out bummed for no real reason? Well, blame low dopamine. It leaves you feeling dull, unexcited, and generally blah. On the flip side, if there's too much dopamine floating around, you might find yourself overly hyped and jittery, almost like you downed one too many coffees. So yeah, it's a balancing act. Your brain depends on dopamine to keep you emotionally on track, and when dopamine goes off course, your mood chases it. Simple as that.

Now, I'm sure you've had those days where ticking off items on your to-do list feels like Herculean tasks. You stare at the list, knowing you need to get stuff done, but **motivation**? Zero. Dopamine steps into play here too. It's your brain's little cheerleader pushing you to go, "Come on, you've got this!" It flushes your brain when anticipating **rewards**—think payday, achieving a goal, or even hitting "send" on a long email. This surge is what gets you moving, firing up your motivation like a car's engine. You see that finish line? Dopamine wants you to get there. But when dopamine's playing hide-and-seek, you end up dragging your feet through the day, everything feeling more like a chore than a challenge.

Ever notice how easily you're distracted when you're supposed to be working on something important? Yep, dopamine is right there in the mix too. You see, dopamine does more than keep you happy and motivated—it's critical for **attention** and **focus**. It's almost like the brain wakes up when dopamine levels are just right, stimulating your focus and sharpening your ability to get stuff done. But when those dopamine levels are off, it's game over for **productivity**. You won't be able to focus on work, reading a book—or even binge-watching a show. Imagine watching a football game, but the crowd noise is distracting you from seeing the key plays—that's your brain on low dopamine.

If your brain's got less dopamine churning through it, your focus drifts. And that zoned-out feeling you get while mindlessly scrolling? Blame dopamine fluctuations for making slumps in attention tougher to snap out of. The next thing you know, you're knee-deep in distractions rather than crushing your to-do list.

To put it all together, mood, motivation, and attention are more connected than you might think, and it all circles back to dopamine. Feeling sad, stuck in **procrastination** like quicksand, or simply unfocused? That could be your brain's way of signaling its dopamine needs a gentle nudge in the right direction.

And there you have it—your brain's little chemical helping hand, giving you all the good vibes, energy, and sharpness you need to tackle the world.

The Dopamine-Reward Connection

You know that **rush** you get when something goes exactly the way you hoped? Well, that's dopamine at work. Think of it like a **reward** system that keeps you coming back for more. There's something called "reward prediction error" that's kind of at the heart of it all. It's this idea that your brain fires off dopamine when the outcome is better or worse than you expected. So, if something good surprises you, bam—you get that hit of dopamine, which leaves you feeling good and wanting more of that action. It's a little bit like playing a slot machine—every time you unexpectedly win, your brain's like, "Let's do that again!" And when the payoff is less than expected? Well, that drop in dopamine levels also sends a message: maybe you don't want to do that again.

But here's the kicker—dopamine doesn't just set off your happy feelings when something good happens. No, it goes way beyond that. Imagine you keep getting that sugar rush from your favorite **candy**. After a while, all it takes is just thinking about it, and voila, your brain already starts releasing dopamine. That's how it nudges you towards actions that bring satisfaction. It's like your brain's little voice saying, "Oh yeah, that was great last time, let's go for it again." You're basically getting rewarded for the thought itself, even before doing anything. Maybe that's why it's so easy to fall back into **habits** that might not always be, well, the best for you. Perfect loop, right?

This leads us to how dopamine plays a tricky role in forming habits. You see something shiny—be it social media, snacks, or a fresh series on Netflix—and dopamine hits you right between the eyes. At first, it's that novelty, that **excitement** of trying something new, or getting into that rabbit hole of cat videos online. But soon, it transforms into full-blown **cravings**. The more you engage, the more dopamine reinforces those patterns, and soon enough, you're not just doing whatever it is because it's simply entertaining anymore. You're like a puppet of your own habits, tugged along by the dopamine strings you yourself have tied.

But... it's not all bad! This system exists for a reason, and it can work for you if you get the wiring right. Imagine using that dopamine loop to create positive routines: working out, learning a language, or even flossing your teeth daily. After all, it's really just about **conditioning**, right? The trick lies in recognizing this loop. And once you do, you're in a better spot to shape what habits stick and which kick the bucket. It's all about small steps and repetitively grabbing the things that serve you, letting dopamine do the rest.

So, this whole dopamine-reward dance is more than just chemical chatter in the brain. It's the **rhythm** that sways you, often without you even noticing. The good news? By understanding how it works, you've got a few tricks up your sleeve for mastering a choreography that won't just take you off-balance, but instead, helps you jump rope with it—step in, step out—while staying in control.

Dopamine's Impact on Decision-Making

Picture yourself standing on the edge of a cliff, **contemplating** whether to leap or back away. That little voice urging you towards the thrill? It might just be **dopamine** whispering in your ear. Known as the "feel-good" chemical, dopamine does more than just boost your mood. It plays a crucial role in whether you take **risks** or play it safe.

When dopamine levels spike, your brain flips a switch, and suddenly, risky decisions seem way more appealing. It's like you've just donned a pair of rose-colored glasses, and everything dangerous starts to look... kinda fun. This can push you to dive into new experiences or try something novel just for the rush—or, on the flip side, it might lead to careless decisions that don't turn out well at all. Your brain is wired to seek out **rewards**, and when it senses a possibility of getting one, dopamine gives you that nudge, making you more likely to roll the dice.

Here's the tricky part: dopamine's also involved in **impulsivity**. The more dopamine pumping through your system, the more you're inclined to act without really thinking through the consequences. That could mean pulling the trigger on that one-click buy online before bedtime... without considering your empty bank account. It's not that dopamine forces you into making rash choices, but it definitely loosens the brakes. It makes the payoff seem closer and the risks far less daunting—even if you're not fully aware of it.

Let's switch gears for a sec and think about how all this impacts your ability to **learn**. Whether you're celebrating a win or licking your wounds after a bad call, your brain's basically taking notes. And dopamine's there, marking out the important bits.

When something happy happens, dopamine gets released. Your brain goes, "Nice, let's do that again!" It helps you remember the good moves and encourages you to stick to strategies that lead to a payoff next time around. That's how you learned that doing a thing well means you're more likely to see a reward again. And, when stuff doesn't go to plan, dopamine's there too—just probably telling you, "Yeah, maybe avoid that."

It's like learning through trial and error. Each win or loss gets tucked away in your brain, and dopamine's basically the highlighter pen pointing your brain in the right direction. But it's not foolproof. A not-so-great experience can sometimes lead to an overdose of caution, reducing your drive to try anything new.

So, what about when you actually need to wait and see if something pays off in the long run? Let me guess, it's not so easy holding out when dopamine's priority is to grab that shiny thing ASAP. When your dopamine levels are pumping, it's tougher to deal with "delayed **gratification**." This means practicing patience or resisting tiny rewards on the way gets tough. Dopamine makes the quicker options seem way more tempting, which might be helpful when instant decisions are needed. But in terms of long-term planning? Not so much.

It's not really about making bad choices, it's about wanting those rewards now, rather than later. Like when you're trying to wake up early tomorrow but end up staying up for "just one more episode." Your brain can get tricked by this rush of dopamine, making it hard to stick to long-term gains when those short-term hits feel so darn good.

So next time you're trying to throttle back on those impulses or stick to a longer plan, just know it's not you—it's your dopamine playing games with your **brain**.

In Conclusion

Dopamine plays a **vital** function in how you feel, think, and act. This chapter explained the essential role of dopamine in your brain, emphasizing how it links to your emotions and **motivates** you to take action. Understanding this complex "chemical messenger" can help you **manage** your emotions and make more mindful decisions.

You've learned that dopamine is a key **neurotransmitter** regulating your brain's reward system. Its levels play a crucial role in controlling your mood and **motivation** levels. Multiple brain regions work together to produce and respond to dopamine. The release of dopamine is closely tied to making decisions, particularly those involving rewards. High or low dopamine can strongly influence your ability to form habits, both good and bad.

Realizing how dopamine can **impact** many parts of your life is the first step toward gaining greater control over your emotions and behaviors. Applying the insights you've gained to your daily life will lead you toward more positive **habits** and better decision-making that can improve the quality of your actions and, ultimately, your overall sense of **well-being**.

Chapter 2: The Dopamine-Driven World

Ever felt like your mind's on **overdrive**, constantly looking for the next hit of excitement? This chapter's gonna dig into why that's happening, and more importantly, what it's doing to you. I've felt that same **rush**—scrolling through endless distractions, searching for that quick fix of pleasure. But do you ever stop and wonder what you're really **trading** for that quick dopamine spike?

As you read, you'll start to question those **habits** you've built, and how they've started to shape your existence. No lectures here, just pointing out the stuff you might've missed while you were caught up in all the **noise**. The goal behind this chapter? Get you thinking about your day-to-day actions, opening up a new kind of **awareness** you didn't even know was possible.

Curious to know what's really going on behind all that stimulation? You're about to find out. This chapter will take you on a journey through the **dopamine**-driven world you're living in, showing you the hidden impacts of your daily choices. You'll start to see how these small decisions are shaping your life in ways you might not have realized.

So buckle up, buddy. You're in for an eye-opening ride that might just change the way you look at your phone, your social media, and pretty much everything else that's vying for your attention. Ready to peek behind the curtain and see what's really pulling the strings? Let's dive in.

Modern Technology and Dopamine Overload

Ever wonder why you can't put your **phone** down or why you keep going back to that one app? It's no accident. Digital **gadgets**—your phone, tablet, or computer—are designed specifically to release dopamine, that sneaky little chemical in your brain that makes you feel good. Thing is, we used to get dopamine hits from food, exercise, even social interactions. But now, these digital gadgets hijack that system, offering you a quicker and more frequent fix.

Every **notification** you get, every like on your latest Instagram post, triggers a small burst of dopamine. Suddenly, your brain is craving more and more of those tiny rewards. It's like training a pet—you get the treat when you behave, so you keep doing it. The problem is, these digital treats come at you nonstop, much faster and more frequent than anything you might have encountered in the past. Suddenly, that next notification becomes the only thing you care about.

Let's dig a little deeper into this. When was the last time you picked up your phone, saw you had a new message, and didn't read it? Even if you were busy, that notification pulled you in, didn't it? What started as a quick check turned into scrolling through an endless **feed** without even realizing it. This is what we call a "dopamine loop." It's this addictive cycle where you keep reaching for the screen, hoping to get that next hit of dopamine. Before you know it, hours have passed, and you've lost yourself in a feed full of other people's updates, cat memes, and food photos.

Dopamine loops aren't by mistake—they're built into the apps themselves. Have you ever noticed how everything looks slightly different but transitional enough to keep you engaged? That's called "variable **rewards**." You never know exactly what you're gonna see, and that unpredictability keeps you glued. Social media platforms, games, even news apps—they're all about keeping you inside that loop.

These loops wouldn't be such a big deal if they were isolated little moments. But they add up fast, changing the way your brain's **reward** system works. It's not just about feeling good anymore; it's about always aiming to meet the next reward level. And you end up stuck in these patterns, where notifications pop up in every quiet moment, whether you want them to or not. Your brain's reward system doesn't get a default reset anymore. It doesn't rest, go hungry, or settle anymore—it's like a marathon runner who never has a finish line. The runner just keeps going and going and going...

Look at how this over-caffeinated connection is messing with your head. When you've constantly got this temptation from social media and apps, it messes hard with how you usually figure out what feels good. Normally, if you do something productive (like completing that task you've been putting off) or something healthy (like going for a jog), the little dopamine gremlins in your brain are all happy to give you a dopamine hit.

Now, with these constant dopamine loops, you might notice that your old stuff just doesn't cut it anymore. What's the point of a quick walk when endlessly swiping gives you rewards quicker? Even worse, these altered reward systems can make everyday life—yes, the real actual things in life—all seem a bit dull in comparison.

So where does that leave you? Well, it messes with everything— from **motivation** to focus. And when your brain rewires itself to chase after short dopamine bursts that add up, real-world things like seeing friends, taking a mindful moment, or doing the meaningful stuff that's genuinely fulfilling—you might start losing interest. There's a whole heap of content out there stopping you from checking in with **reality**, and that's rewiring how your brain deals with reward entirely.

Seems like a treadmill from which there's no getting off.

Social Media and the Dopamine Loop

Ever notice how hard it is to put your phone down sometimes? Like **scrolling** just has you hooked, and you can't even explain why? Yeah, it's not just you. Social media platforms are designed to be addictive. It's not a coincidence; it's their whole business model. They know you're more likely to stay engaged as long as you keep getting satisfied. You see, when you open an app and start scrolling, you're actually sparking a reaction in your brain's reward system, kinda like when you eat your favorite dessert. But what keeps you coming back is even sneakier than that.

Let's look at how this works. You might hit the refresh button every so often, right? Every time you do, your brain gears up for a potential reward. Might be that someone liked your post or maybe commented. Maybe they didn't, but that slight chance is good enough to keep you scrolling. That's no accident. It's those "what if" moments that send your brain spinning. When you do get a **notification**, your brain gets a little shot of **dopamine**—a chemical that makes you feel good—for a second. But here's the thing: because you don't always get those rewards, you end up craving them more. And there you are, lost in endless scrolling... chasing a feeling that comes and goes.

These platforms are more than just simple communication tools. They're built to play with your emotions, mostly through something called "unpredictable rewards."

In simpler terms, "unpredictable rewards" are like dangling a carrot in front of your brain but never knowing when you'll get to eat it. Social media **algorithms** are designed to sprinkle in these surprises just enough to keep you engaged—but not constantly. So, the big hit for your brain doesn't come from knowing you'll get rewarded but rather from not knowing. It's an ancient trick, really. Your brain is wired to seek out pleasure and avoid pain, and it's always on the lookout for the next little boost of joy. This system is so hardwired that even if you don't get that "hit" right away—you're primed to try again. Scroll. Maybe this time you'll find something interesting. You don't, but then—out of the blue—you come across a hilarious meme or an unexpected notification. Boom! Dopamine fills your brain, telling you, "Hey, that felt good. Let's do it again." See the loop forming here?

So, imagine that constant grabbing for likes, comments, or shares. We've talked about the "why," but it's crucial to get into the "how." How are your dopamine levels getting yanked around the minute you log in? That's the third ingredient in this cocktail—**social validation**.

The idea here is pretty simple, but oh-so-effective. When people "like" your post or leave a comment, they're basically saying, "You belong. You're important." That sense of social approval or acceptance feels amazing—so amazing, in fact, that it sends your dopamine levels soaring higher than before. That's when things start to get messy. One like leads to "Was that enough? Maybe I should post more..." and before long, your nights are spent polishing that perfect Instagram caption or crafting that viral TikTok. Your brain keeps hoping for another ding of satisfaction. And this process? The cycle can wear you out emotionally, almost without you noticing. Your mind craves more; it's wired that way. And social platforms? Well, they know it all too well.

All in all, social media doesn't just tap into your brain's **reward system**—it's more like it **hijacks** it. Keeping you hooked is no accident; in fact, it's kind of the point.

Instant Gratification Culture

You live in a world where getting things quick ain't just convenient—it's something you've come to **expect**. Want some food? Order it online and it's at your door within minutes. Need a new gadget? Same-day delivery. Everything's instant—just a few clicks away. But this isn't only making life easier. It's also messing with your **dopamine** system. Every time you refresh your social media app and see a 'like' pop up, your brain loves it, gives you that good old rush of dopamine. But that quick hit? It's not helping in the long run. It's more like you're chasing a high, one that's more about the moment than anything real or lasting.

When your brain gets used to these easy, fast **rewards**, it starts to crave them. You might notice that you're beginning to want things more quickly, and getting impatient when they don't come immediately. That's what instant **gratification** does—it kills your patience. Like when you're waiting for someone to text you back, and every minute feels like an hour. Or think about this: how do you feel when you're stuck in traffic scrolling through a feed that isn't updating? The itchiness, the need to see something new… it's all part of how this craving develops. You get so used to everything being instant, that the slightly slower stuff—like waiting in line or even reading an entire book—becomes almost unbearable. It's frustrating because your brain, and that restless dopamine of yours, would rather have the quick fix instead.

So, what happens when you keep churning through these rapid hits of dopamine again and again? Well, over time, you might find out that it's affecting more than just your mood; it's tweaking how you approach the bigger things in life. Imagine you're saving for something nice, like a vacation or a new car. If you're constantly satisfying your need—by going for all the small stuff that immediately strokes your dopamine—it suddenly makes waiting for that something real, something that takes **patience**, so much harder. It becomes challenging to deal with the longer waits, 'cause your brain's been trained towards looking for the fast fix, always prioritizing the short-term over real, lasting gratification.

Now if you think about it, if you're always grabbing at those quick flashes—social media likes, instant movies, or those 10-minute meals—you're kind of robbing yourself of the joy that comes from things that take time. That vacation after months of saving? Now it kinda feels less gratifying, less enjoyable. So getting stuck in the habit of choosing the instant reward every single time—'cause it's easier and right there—means you're missing out on the things that require more **effort** but return so much more **satisfaction**. It's like the difference between splurging on fast food every day versus waiting in excitement, anticipation for a meal you really deserve and savoring it… Well, the impact of too much instant gratification can stretch beyond just your drive-thru decisions; it can creep into other parts of your life too.

That's why it's good to ask yourself—a quick hit or something worth waiting for? If you train your brain to only deal with the 'right now,' you might just find that it loses the ability to tough it out for something **awesome** that's just a little farther down the road.

The Downside of Constant Stimulation

Your **brain** is like a muscle. You work it out with every new piece of information, every notification, every scroll through social media. But when muscles are overstretched, they get tired—and worse, they don't grow as strong. The same thing can happen to your brain, especially when it comes to **dopamine**. See, dopamine's that little burst of happiness and pleasure your brain gives you when something exciting happens. It's your brain's way of rewarding you. But if you're always chasing those rewards, that rush of dopamine doesn't work the way it should.

Here's the thing: when you're constantly overstimulated, your dopamine system ends up overwhelmed. Imagine trying to focus while five different conversations are happening around you. Over time, brains that are bombarded with too much stimulation—like through phones, games, social events—don't get the same thrill from it anymore. You start needing more and more to hit that same level. It's like a rollercoaster that you were once really excited to ride. The first few times, it's exhilarating. But after plummeting down that same drop over and over, suddenly it's not doing it for you anymore—you want a bigger, faster, more intense rush.

This leads us straight into a little something called "**hedonic adaptation**." Here's how it works: when you constantly seek out pleasure, your brain adapts by wanting more intense experiences to feel that same satisfaction. It's like trying to quench your thirst with a few sips of water, but only getting thirstier. Pretty soon, the simple joys—like sitting on a quiet porch at dawn, feeling the sun warm your face—don't have the same appeal.

You might have noticed this happening in your own life. Gotten caught up refreshing your social media or binge-watching a show, but afterwards, found that things you used to enjoy felt kind of dull. That's how hedonic adaptation sneaks up on you. What was thrilling becomes something predictable and, well, boring. And like I said earlier, the more you feed it, the hungrier it gets.

But there's a bigger challenge—following that constant need for **stimulation** can mess with your mind in other ways, too. Guess what? Research suggests that being overstimulated can be strongly connected to **anxiety** and **depression**. You know that feeling of restlessness you have after spending too much time flicking through your phone at night? It's your mind stuck in a loop of wanting more info, more excitement, but the shiny stuff you consume just leaves you more jittery or down. Think of it as ramping up your brain's speed without really going anywhere.

Here's the scary part: overstimulation stops you from savoring the quieter, simpler moments in life. Where normally some sunshine or a walk in the park might have soothed you, overstimulation can actually make calmness feel unbearable. Your mind's barely had a chance to rest, so it goes on strike. Your dopamine is demanding something bigger and better—or nothing feels right, and you're left with that anxiety that has no clear cause. Brains evolved to handle the quiet alongside the noise. A balanced back-and-forth. When you push too much on the "on" side of things, that's when anxiety crawls back in.

And whether you realize it or not, being depressed often involves longing for something just out of your reach or feeling strangely emotionless, even toward things you once loved. There's literally nothing exciting anymore—not because life's changed, but because you overloaded those happy circuits. Your pastimes, your hobbies, all that extra attention—it was kind of like having too much ice cream and not tasting the flavors with each spoonful.

In simple terms? It's about appreciating not overloading. Kicking a habit of constant stimulation could mean enjoying things like a sunrise or a simple conversation with a friend again—without needing extra prompts or distractions or drawn-out highs. Just pure, uncomplicated **contentment**—and trust me, that's worth making those moments count.

In Conclusion

This chapter sheds light on the **significant** role dopamine plays in your daily life, particularly how modern technology has created a dopamine-driven world where instant gratification prevails. Understanding these concepts can help guide you in **managing** your interaction with technology more effectively.

You've seen how technology creates constant dopamine triggers. Your phone, apps, and online platforms are **designed** to keep you hooked by continuously stimulating your brain's reward system. You've learned about the impact of "dopamine loops" - these instant reward cycles that keep you coming back to your devices, which can lead to habitual and potentially **addictive** behavior.

The effects of constant connectivity have been **explored**. Always being connected can overwhelm your brain, affecting how you perceive rewards and making you less satisfied in the long run. You've discovered the link between social media and dopamine release. Each like, share, or comment provides a quick, but temporary, spike of happiness that can turn into a never-ending loop of seeking **validation** online.

The downside of instant gratification has been highlighted. Constant quick rewards can make it harder to appreciate and **work** towards long-term fulfillment, impacting your motivation and overall happiness.

As you reflect on these points, consider how your current **habits** surrounding technology and instant gratification might be shaping your life. Now's the time to apply the lessons learned, make healthier choices, and take control of your dopamine-driven actions for a more balanced and fulfilling lifestyle.

Chapter 3: The Pleasure-Pain Balance

Imagine if you could finally make sense of that constant **tug-of-war** between pleasure and pain. Wouldn't life feel more manageable? I've been there, wrestling with why some things feel amazing until, well, they suddenly don't. That's what this chapter's all about—figuring out how to regain your footing in this **balancing act**.

You've probably noticed how the pursuit of a little pleasure can tip the scales into a kind of strange discomfort, right? You might wonder—why is it so darn hard to keep things **balanced**? In this chapter, I'll walk you through what's really going on in your **brain**—the part where **dopamine** steps in and tries to take control. But don't worry, we're not just diving into the chaos, we're sorting through it. By the end, you'll have the **tools** to find the balance again.

Ever felt like you're on a rollercoaster of highs and lows? That's your **pleasure-pain** system at work. It's like your brain's built-in DJ, always trying to mix the perfect track of feel-good vibes and necessary caution. Sometimes it nails it, and other times, well, let's just say the remix needs work.

You're about to get the inside scoop on how this internal DJ operates. We'll dive into why that extra slice of pizza feels so good in the moment but leaves you feeling like a stuffed turkey later. Or why scrolling through social media can be so addictive, even when you know you should be hitting the hay.

Ready to crack the code of your own pleasure-pain **balance**? Let's jump in and unravel this mystery together. By the time we're done, you'll be the master of your own internal equilibrium. Buckle up, buddy—it's going to be one heck of a ride!

The Neuroscience of Pleasure and Pain

You might not realize it, but **pleasure** and **pain** are deeply intertwined in your brain. When you experience something enjoyable—like savoring your favorite dessert or receiving a spot-on compliment—it's not just random. These feelings are actually connected to the possibility of discomfort. Sounds weird, right? It's as if these two sensations are constantly duking it out in your head.

Picture yourself at a party, grooving to your favorite tunes—pure **bliss**. But there's that nagging thought lurking in the back of your mind, isn't there? The one that whispers about tomorrow's gloomy hangover and throbbing headache. That's pain, sneaking up when you least expect it. Your brain links pleasure and pain through the same **reward** system. When you feel good, your brain releases dopamine, that feel-good chemical that makes you crave more. But here's the kicker: it's not unlimited. The more dopamine you release, the more your brain has to balance things out, leading to a kind of letdown once that high fades away.

So, how does this stuff actually work? Imagine your **emotions** are controlled by two opposing forces in your brain. On one side, you've got pleasure; on the other, pain. Your brain's constantly trying to keep things balanced. It's like standing on one foot—with every little sway to one side, you desperately try to move the other way to stay upright. In brain terms, this means that whenever you feel a surge of pleasure, your brain anticipates a dive towards the pain side to even things out.

Yeah, it sounds pretty intense because it is. There's even a clever name for this see-saw situation—opponent-process theory. Not too flashy, but it drives home the point that emotions move like a pendulum. When they swing too far on the pleasure side, they'll almost always swing back to equal things out. That's why devouring a box of chocolates at midnight might make you feel warm inside, but hours later? You're regretting that sugar crash. It's your brain doing its typical balancing act.

But hey, there's more cool stuff happening inside your head. While dopamine hogs a lot of the spotlight when it comes to pleasure, there are other important chemicals you shouldn't forget. Think of them as background characters with major roles. Take **serotonin**, for instance; it's the chemical that helps keep your mood stable, preventing you from tipping too far over to the painful side. Ever noticed how biting into that juicy piece of fruit makes you content in an entirely different way? That's serotonin in action. It doesn't give you the immediate, intense euphoria like dopamine does, but it works behind the scenes to keep you from toppling into anxiety or sadness.

And wait... there's still **endorphins**. These little guys are like your brain's natural painkillers. When you get hurt or, say, run a marathon, endorphins come swooping in to mask the pain, tricking you into feeling pretty amazing afterward instead. They share the stage with dopamine but work in opposite ways. Imagine dopamine as fireworks in the sky while endorphins are the calm sunrise that fills you with quiet satisfaction instead of blaring excitement. Different but crucial.

So, when you take it all in, what you're really dealing with is a brain full of chemical scales. Lean too much one way, and your brain will shift things around to keep your world from tipping over. Whether it's handling that dopamine rush or cushioning you with serotonin and endorphins, your brain's got a method to its madness. It's all there in the **balance** between pleasure and pain—helping you feel alive and sort of keeping you grounded along the way, crazy as that may sound.

Dopamine's Role in the Balance

You've probably heard that dopamine is like the "feel-good" chemical. And sure, there's some truth to that. But it isn't just about triggering **pleasure** each time you bite into a slice of pizza or get a like on your social media post. There's more going on beneath the surface when it comes to dopamine—and life isn't always just about feeling great. It's about balancing between pleasure and **pain**. Yep, dopamine has a role in that too.

Imagine dopamine as a **signal**, one that helps you figure out what to pay attention to in your life. It's not just rewarding your brain with good feelings for the heck of it—dopamine is really marking out what your brain decides is important. This means it gives a nudge when you're on the brink of doing something that could pay off in one way or another. It's kind of like how a teacher gives you a gold star for the effort, but inside your body.

But just like a teacher who gives out too many gold stars until they don't mean anything anymore, dopamine can mess you up when it's out of whack. If your dopamine is all over the place, that steady signal can turn into noise, making your brain misfire about what's really important. Feeling too much dopamine too often can even tip the scales on how you feel pain. Suddenly, little things bother you way more—because with everything in overdrive, your sense of **balance** gets disrupted.

That misfire? It's like a shift from being tuned into life's pleasures to feeling pain more intensely. When that happens, maybe you turn to things—like food, screens, or even drugs to try to feel good again—even for just a bit. Dopamine's high, followed by the inevitable low, can keep you running around, looking for that next "hit," even when it's not good for you. It's less about the pleasure you're trying to get and more about avoiding pain. A sort of down escalator where things feel heavier the further you go.

Now this skewed **sensitivity**? It's why many folks end up addicted. Ever notice how someone addicted will start chasing the thing, whether drugs, games, or junk food, not even to feel pleasure anymore? It's more about making the constant nagging pain or discomfort go away. But every time you try the "feel good" route to drown the discomfort, your brain just builds up tolerance, meaning you'll need more of whatever brings that rush, while your pain thresholds keep on messing with you.

So, really, it's not about simply "more dopamine means more pleasure." Balance matters. Think of it like Ariana's "The Light is Coming," only this time, it takes away the good things too if you're not careful. And that's the real trick this tricky **neurotransmitter** plays. Balanced levels will help guide you through and help you focus on what's really meaningful—sending you nudges that matter, but not blowing up into making you feel twists of too high then way too low.

You gotta keep that pleasure-pain balance in check, watching it like you'd keep an eye on the simmering pot making your favorite stew. If you're careful with it, you'll end up in a better place where pleasures don't drive you to the brink and pain doesn't keep you in its hold. Too much of anything? It's a recipe for **trouble**—dopamine included—leaving you chasing that uncontrollable see-saw, rather than contenting yourself in the in-between.

Tolerance and Adaptation

Let's talk about how your **brain** just gets used to things. You know that feeling when you start a new **hobby**, eat your favorite ice cream, or hear a song you can't stop humming? At first, it's all super exciting. But over time, that feeling fades a bit. Why? It's not because you love it any less. It's because your brain has started to get used to it. This is what scientists call **tolerance** and **adaptation**. Honestly, your brain is like that too-inflated balloon. At first, just a little push can blow your mind. But push it repeatedly? It takes more to get the same rush.

Here's how it works: when you first try something that releases **dopamine**—like eating that perfect chocolate or getting a like on social media—boom! Your brain lights up like a Christmas tree. You feel totally satisfied. But if you keep eating that chocolate or scrolling through posts, the brain starts to adjust. It kind of says, "Oh, we've seen this before. Not as thrilling anymore." So next time, you need even more chocolate or even more likes to feel that same high. And the crazy part? If you keep pushing it, your brain starts getting lazy at producing dopamine naturally.

This doesn't just happen with good stuff—it's the same with the bad too. Ever stubbed your toe real badly? At the moment, it's unbearable. But if you're in constant **pain**, let's say with a chronic issue, your brain starts to dull that pain over time. It doesn't completely go away, but you become somewhat numb, more tolerant of the pain. The brain, for survival's sake, says, "Okay, I've got this under control now, nothing new here."

So, what does all this mean for you, especially if you're dealing with something like **addiction** or constant pain? Well, it's tough. Like, really tough. With addiction, your brain craves more and more of that dopamine hit because it's adapted to the usual amount. You end up chasing that high, often sinking into harmful habits. It's a vicious cycle because no matter how much more you get, it's never quite enough. At a certain point, your brain is so desensitized that the things that once made you happy or content hardly make a dent in your mood anymore. Now you're left in a place where your brain is searching for moments of pleasure and is avoiding the lows, and, because it's always adapting—that balance skews big time.

For chronic pain or addiction, this tolerance and adaptation piece is downright crucial. You see, your brain tries to deal with things by building up tolerance. In doing that, it demands even more extremes—either of pleasure or pain relief. Short-term, it seems helpful. Long-term? Not so much. In a weird way, your own brain does this to protect you initially but ends up making things more challenging.

In the end, your brain gets stuck in this loop, constantly trying to find **equilibrium**. Whether you're battling addiction, or learning to manage chronic pain, it's like being on a seesaw, trying to balance out that pleasure-pain teeter-totter where tolerance keeps shifting the fulcrum. The more you push, the more the balance tips everywhere except where you want it. It's much like inflating a balloon where, after a while, it takes more effort to get that same thrill. This is why awareness and understanding are critical—don't get tricked by your own dopamine game.

Restoring Equilibrium

Ever notice how your **brain** has a way of balancing things out? It's like a natural scale that weighs good stuff against the bad stuff. When you grab a taste of something nice—like chocolate, binge-watching your favorite show, or smashing through a workout—your brain gets its hit of **dopamine**. That's what gives you that rush of pleasure.

But your brain's pretty smart. It knows not to let things get out of hand. Because too much of a good thing can backfire. So when that hit of dopamine comes in, your brain releases chemicals that push the scale back. These chemicals swing the needle toward pain or discomfort to level things out. Imagine running a marathon. That runner's high starts to wear off, and then... boom, you're exhausted. That's your brain trying to keep everything in check—showing you that it's not all thrills and triumphs. So the brain's always on this teeter-totter, balancing **pleasure** with pain, adjusting to keep everything in equilibrium. It's an ongoing tug-of-war, really.

Now when things change or stick around long-term, your body starts to play along. If you've ever had a long streak of **stress**—maybe a tough work period or a rough patch—it can start to feel normal. Like you're used to it. Same story with rewards—say you've been getting a treat every Friday for months. The high you used to get? It's not as strong. Your brain kind of adjusts to that regular dose. This is **adaptation** in action. It's your brain's way of not overloading the grid.

When you're swimming in stress for weeks, your body starts making tweaks to stay functional. The stress hasn't gone away, you've just settled into it. You adjust along the way, but there's a price. Maybe your energy dips, or your nerves get a little more touchy. It's a give-and-take...and your body wants to make sure you don't crumble under the pressure.

The same holds when you level up your pleasure: your brain tones down the vibe, pulling it back from the highs so they don't completely burn you out. It's like you've built up a resistance—an immunity, if you like. Unfortunately, the downside kicks in, too. The stuff that used to leave you ecstatic now just leaves you feeling 'meh.' It's your brain trying to keep a steady course, resisting the urge to get too hooked on anything, whether it's a thrill or a pain.

The beauty is, your brain knows how to reset that system. You can retrain your dopamine hit with the simple trick of changing your **habits**. Maybe by tweaking your fun—like mixing up rewards—or by tackling harmful streaks of stress and shaking up the rut you've dug yourself into. Your brain stretches and adjusts because it's pretty good at knowing when things are out of whack. An easy swap can shift your mindset. Instead of a screen snack, take a short walk. Instead of clinging to spirals of tension, unplug with deep breaths. These small moves nudge your brain to reset the scales, inching you toward **balance** quicker than you'd expect.

So leaning into new activities and cutting those bad loops is the secret formula to letting your system recover. Cozying up to these tiny changes awards you good vibes, lifting you slowly out of energy slumps or grinding down that constant stress mountain, so the brain cops a better balance. It's the brainman's way of fixing its own ship, steering it toward calmer seas.

In Conclusion

This chapter has given you a **fascinating glimpse** into how your brain handles pleasure and pain, showing how your emotional experiences are shaped by specific neurological processes. The interplay between these two sensations highlights the delicate and **complex nature** of your mental equilibrium, especially when it comes to your brain's chemistry. A key focus was on dopamine, which isn't just a harbinger of joy but a **crucial regulator** of various states, including pain.

You've learned that your brain processes pleasure and pain in tandem, balancing these sensations through intricate mechanisms. Dopamine plays a **significant role** in how you experience both delight and discomfort. It's much more than just a "happiness chemical."

Your brain can sometimes get used to certain feelings, leading to tolerance. This can be a **tricky issue** with addiction or chronic pain. Your brain constantly tries to maintain equilibrium even when pleasure or pain signals shift, but this adjustment period can have **long-lasting effects**.

The good news is that it's possible to **alter how** your brain processes pleasure and pain. This opens up opportunities for recovery from addiction or better coping with chronic stress.

By applying what you've read, you can **transform your perspective** on emotional experiences. Understanding the dynamics of pleasure and pain in your brain empowers you to manage your feelings more effectively and work towards a more balanced, healthier life.

Chapter 4: Recognizing Dopamine Imbalance

Ever felt like your **moods** are on a rollercoaster, and you're just along for the ride? I've been there, too. This chapter takes you on a bit of a journey into how our favorite chemical, **dopamine**, can either be your best friend or a bit of a troublemaker. You might want to tap into something familiar—those days when getting off the couch feels impossible or when **focusing** on a task seems like the hardest thing in the world. If you've wondered "Why?", this chapter might give you some clues.

You're not just learning for curiosity's sake here; you're figuring out how to get **control** back. As you go through this, you're not just reading words—you're grabbing onto something that could change how you **feel** day to day. It's about understanding those times when your **motivation** seems to have taken a vacation or when your **energy** levels are all over the place.

This chapter isn't just about recognizing the signs of dopamine imbalance; it's about **empowering** yourself with knowledge. You'll start to see patterns in your behavior and moods that you might not have noticed before. It's like putting on a pair of glasses and suddenly seeing everything in sharper focus.

So, buckle up and get ready to dive into the world of dopamine. By the end of this chapter, you'll have a better grasp on what makes you tick and how to keep your internal **chemistry** working in your favor. Trust me, it's going to be an eye-opener!

Indicators of Dopamine Deficiency

You **wake** up feeling exhausted, drag yourself to your first cup of coffee, and things don't get much better from there. Sound familiar? It might not just be a rough day. That dragging, unmotivated feeling could be a sign of something deeper, like low dopamine. You're bound to run into this if you don't get your chemical balance sorted out.

So what does dopamine have to do with feeling like you'll never be selling vacation packages with your sparkling **energy** and charisma? A lot, actually. Dopamine is a chemical that your brain relies on to fire up, like needing decent gas for your car. Feeling sluggish, like you didn't get the memo on what's keeping everyone else motivated? That's likely because dopamine's missing from the party.

And it's not just about feeling lazy. You need dopamine to feel **pleasure** too, so when your tank's empty, everything from books to hobbies starts to seem kind of... meh. You might have to drag yourself through things you once loved. The buzz? Gone. Remember when you binged on a series and didn't mind the usual dull thudding heartbeat of life? With low dopamine, that zest slips away—fast.

Keep in mind, dopamine doesn't only affect enjoyment and drive; it sneaks into nearly everything you do. When your reserve is too low, watch out. Suddenly, staying **optimistic** or managing your emotions gets trickier, and you don't want to stay stuck in a joyless fog, right? You might find yourself spending more time feeling irritated by the smallest things or snapping at those you usually adore. It's a bit like someone put a sour lens on your outlook.

But low dopamine doesn't just make small tasks seem like mountains; it pulls the emotional rug out as well. What used to inspire or lighten your **mood** now comes with a side of indifference, isolating you emotionally from stuff and people who matter most.

Have you ever walked into your favorite place only to feel nothing, though nothing has changed? That flatline in mood isn't just moodiness—it's chemistry. You're messaging more in your head, guessing that was dopamine slipping away, honestly wondering if you can stop losing the one thing that kept your energy fueling happiness.

Between sinking **energy** levels and losing a passion for things, there's one more aspect where dopamine deficiency shows up wearing the signs: your habits. That feeling of sliding into poor routines? Yep, blame dopamine. When it's low, you're less likely to maintain healthy habits or push through the usual challenges because—it's almost like a switch in your brain skips that "feeling good after task completion" stage. So you opt for what feels easier. Maybe you lose hours scrolling through your phone, or obsessively snack even when you're not hungry—anything to get that meager dopamine trickle going. But they aren't long-term solutions, they're signs of depletion, clear as day.

Which brings us to something practical: How do you know if dopamine is the root of the **trouble** in your life? Here's a helpful list to consider—all symptoms that can be connected to low dopamine. But don't check these too quickly, yeah?

• Feeling perpetually tired, even after restful sleep

• Finding it hard to get started on any activities

• Losing interest in things that once made you happy

• Difficulty managing stress or becoming easily frustrated

• Eating easily pleasurable foods, even when you're not hungry

• Struggling with focus, always distracted

If you checked "yes" more than once, well, dopamine deficiency might be affecting you more than you think. The great news? Once you start paying attention to tracking these potential imbalances, you can actually aim (in a holistic manner, of course) at restoring your **energy** and passion levels. It's action, not just awareness, that's future-success fuel.

Symptoms of Dopamine Excess

Too much of a good thing can become a problem—especially when it comes to **dopamine**. When dopamine is too high, it doesn't just give you energy and motivation—it can start to push you into overdrive. And that overdrive? Well, that's where you might start noticing some changes in your behavior that aren't exactly doing you any favors.

You might find yourself making decisions a little too quickly, saying "yes" before you fully think things through. That's **impulsiveness**, plain and simple. It can be something as small as buying yet another gadget because it looks cool, or as big as jumping into a risky business venture without really considering if it's worth it. This impulsive behavior isn't just about being a little too enthusiastic—it's a straight-up red flag that your dopamine levels might be on the high side. When your brain is flooded with dopamine, it pushes you to keep seeking that next rush, that next hit of excitement. But the problem isn't just that you're chasing thrills; it's that you might stop caring about the consequences.

And while we're on the topic of chasing highs, let's talk about **risk-taking**. Yep, dopamine can turn you into a bit of a daredevil. Whether it's making bold investments you wouldn't normally consider or deciding to take up a new hobby that's pretty dangerous, an excess of dopamine can crank up your willingness to take chances. Sure, a little risk can be fun and even rewarding, but when you're consistently choosing the risky route without much thought to the downsides, it's a sign something's off in your brain's balance. So if you're noticing yourself diving headfirst into things that, in the clearer light of day, make you shake your head—check in with those dopamine levels.

Now, impulsiveness and risk-taking are issues on their own, but they also have a way of spilling over into your bigger life decisions and how you handle your **emotions**. When dopamine's got you wired, you may start to notice that you're not making the best choices when it comes to important decisions. Suppose you're so focused on that quick payoff that you forget to think about the bigger picture—or that your fiery temper flares more often than you'd like. It's not just about making rash decisions or being more easily swayed; it's also about feeling like you're on an emotional rollercoaster. Those highs and lows can be much more intense when dopamine's driving the car, leaving you overwhelmed or even snapping at others without meaning to.

So how do you know if too much dopamine is really the culprit? Well, you might need to check yourself with a "**Dopamine Excess Self-Assessment**." Think about your recent behavior and decisions. Are you saying "yes" to things on the fly? Are you drawn to risks you wouldn't normally take? Are your emotions running a little wild? If any—or all—of these ring a bell, you might be looking at a dopamine imbalance. Keeping tabs on yourself through such an assessment can help you identify if these patterns are getting out of hand.

One way to do a short self-check could look something like this:

• Do you often make snap decisions and regret them later?

• Are you drawn to risky activities, despite knowing the dangers?

• Do you feel like your emotions are more intense or unchecked than usual?

Answering "yes" to these questions could suggest you've got a bit too much dopamine running through your system. Recognizing these **signs** is just the first step—the next one is figuring out how to bring things back to a more balanced state.

So, if you've been feeling more scattered, risky, or emotionally charged than usual, it's time to pause and reflect. Not only will understanding these **symptoms** help bring you back into balance, but it'll also keep you from spinning out of control.

The Connection Between Dopamine and Mental Health

You've probably had those days when **motivation** seems to vanish into thin air, no matter how hard you try. It might feel like it's just "one of those days," but there's actually more going on behind the scenes. It all comes down to a tiny but **powerful** neurotransmitter called dopamine. This chemical isn't just about giving you a good buzz now and then; it's intimately linked to your mood, focus, and overall **mental health**.

Let's start with feeling down—because who hasn't been there? When your brain's dopamine levels are out of whack, it can hit you right in the feels, making you **struggle** with sadness or emptiness. If levels drop too low, it's like someone's dimmed all the lights on your emotional control panel. It's not just in your head either; dopamine imbalances have been linked to conditions like depression. So if your dopamine isn't playing ball, it's no wonder that just getting out of bed feels like lifting a boulder. You're not just tired; the spark that's supposed to fuel your drive is flickering.

But hold up—there's more to the story. Low dopamine levels can mess with your **focus** too. Ever sat down to work or study and found your mind wandering or feeling foggy? Wonky dopamine can turn your brain into a distracted mess. This trouble concentrating can be tied to disorders like ADHD, where people constantly struggle to focus, even when they really want to.

Here's the kicker—dopamine isn't just about fueling moods and focus. It plays a sneaky role in **addiction** too. Ever wondered why it's so easy to get hooked on things like social media, junk food, or even shopping? It all ties back to dopamine giving you that "just one more" feeling that pushes you to repeat behaviors. When your mind gets that dopamine rush from checking your phone (or, let's be real, watching another cat video), it wants you to do it again—pronto. You might not even enjoy the habit anymore. What you're hooked on is that tiny dopamine kick. Unfortunately, that "fix" can leave you feeling trapped, doing things that aren't even fun, just because your brain's chasing that expected hit.

Now, picture this as a mental health maze. Start with dopamine at the top, then draw arrows pointing to conditions like depression, ADHD, and addiction. For each of these, add lines to related **symptoms**—like lack of motivation, poor focus, or repetitive behaviors. A messed-up dopamine level doesn't just trigger one condition; it often causes a domino effect that impacts multiple areas of your life.

Put it all together, and what have you got? Dopamine is like this hidden master switch in your brain, controlling your mental health without you even realizing it. When it's balanced, everything runs smoothly. But when levels go haywire? The whole system can come crashing down, and if you're not clued in, it's easy to mistake those symptoms as isolated problems rather than pieces of the same dopamine-related puzzle.

This knowledge is crucial because understanding the dopamine connection could be like realizing you've been playing life on hard mode all along. Once you grasp how it all fits together, you might just find the cheat codes to level up your mental health game.

Evaluating Your Dopamine Levels

Alright, so you might be wondering how to tell if your dopamine levels are actually out of whack. It's not like you're equipped with mood meters that beep when something's off. But here's the thing— you don't need a fancy test to spot patterns in your behavior that signal issues. The clues are there, you've just got to know where to look.

Let's talk about those patterns. What do you notice about your thinking and behavior when everything's good? You feel **motivated**, probably more social, maybe even pumped to tackle tasks. But if dopamine isn't balanced, things start to waver. You could feel "blah" at times when you'd expect to feel excited. Or on the flip side, maybe you feel super charged—and not in a great way. Acting **impulsively**, chasing high energy all the time but wearing yourself out... that's your brain needing a break. And heads-up, chasing short-term "wins" like binge-eating, social media, or thrill-seeking could be a huge red flag. Dopamine imbalance is sort of like someone messing with your mix—a little too much of one thing, not enough of another.

Are there situations where you feel more alive or like you're dragging your feet? Start noting them. It's these little shifts that really clue you in on when your brain **chemistry** isn't working to your advantage. Are certain tasks always boring no matter how much rest you get? Or maybe you find yourself ducking out of social events you used to love. Jot that down. The trick is finding a pattern, something that doesn't really change whether you're well-rested or stressed.

Sometimes it's easy to miss these clues. You might not notice how your **motivation** waxes and wanes. But tracking them is like looking through a collage over time. Every small observation adds up. Which is exactly why you should start keeping a "mood radar" (let's be fancy and call it the "Daily Dopamine Diary"). Doesn't need to be anything too serious; just grab a notebook and try documenting what you did, how you felt, and your energy level as the day goes on. Need an afternoon pick-me-up? Note it. Felt like

procrastination was running your life today? Note it. Scroll through Instagram for an hour instead of sending that email? Put it in the Diary.

Now, not every "off" day will scream dopamine imbalance, but all those dips and spikes over days or weeks will show patterns. Maybe you're always **motivated** on Saturday mornings but fall into a slump by nighttime. Or maybe hitting social media at lunch is your go-to dopamine pick-me-up. Whatever you find, this systematic tracking helps nail down what drives your **behavior** and mood. Over time, you'll see it; you'll know when something throws your dopamine spirals.

So take control—start listening to how you truly feel, even in those little daily moments. That's how you spot when your **dopamine** is working either too much... or not enough. Then, your brain's behavior "mix" won't surprise you at every single turn.

In Conclusion

This chapter has shed light on how **dopamine** imbalances can significantly impact your **mood** and **behaviors**. Recognizing these imbalances, understanding the **symptoms** associated with both deficits and excesses, and taking active steps to evaluate your own dopamine levels can be key in leading a more balanced life. By paying attention to the clues your body and mind give you, you can make smarter choices to improve your **mental health**.

You've learned about the telltale signs that might indicate a possible dopamine deficiency, such as a lack of **energy** and struggling to enjoy life. You've also discovered types of behavior that could signify you've got more dopamine than you need, including impulsiveness and overreacting to small problems. These imbalances are linked to conditions like depression or ADHD, highlighting the importance of regularly observing your daily actions, moods, and feelings to help identify what triggers these unbalanced states.

The chapter has emphasized the value of tracking how your mood, **motivation**, and habits intersect with your dopamine levels to get a clearer picture of your mental well-being. It's all about connecting the dots between what you're experiencing and what's going on inside your brain.

Making small adjustments and being mindful can go a long way in managing your dopamine levels better. The more you pay attention now, the more in **control** you can be later on. So, keep an eye on those mood swings, energy levels, and daily habits – they're your personal barometer for dopamine balance. Remember, it's not about perfection, but about understanding yourself better and making informed choices for your mental health.

Chapter 5: The Science of Dopamine Regulation

Have you ever **wondered** why some days you feel on top of the world, while others leave you dragging your feet through molasses? I know that feeling too—like you're trying to untangle a mess of tightly knotted cords and all you find is more confusion. Well, this chapter is here to untangle some of those knots for you. We're going to chat about what's **happening** inside your **brain** that makes those swings happen.

It'll become clearer how your brain **wires** itself to these hits and misses, what tips the scales, and how to balance things out. There's a kind of **balance** happening—and when it's just right, things just click. But there's more... ever felt **stress** wreak havoc on your fun, like a raincloud spoiling a parade? We'll talk about that too.

Trust me, by the end you'll have lots more **figured** out. Just keep reading, and you'll gain a better **understanding** of how your brain works. You might even start to see patterns in your own behavior that you never noticed before. It's like putting on a pair of glasses for the first time—suddenly, everything comes into focus.

So buckle up, buddy. We're about to dive into the fascinating world of dopamine regulation. It might sound complicated, but I promise to break it down in a way that'll make sense to you. Who knows? You might even find yourself explaining this stuff to your friends at your next hangout. Let's get started, shall we?

Neuroplasticity and Dopamine

Have you ever wondered how your **brain** manages to stay so adaptable throughout your life? It's all thanks to something called **neuroplasticity**. It's basically the brain's superpower, the ability to change and rewire itself over time. Think of it like learning to ride a bike as a kid—it feels wobbly at first, but after a few attempts, your brain gets the hang of it, adjusting and building new pathways so your body works with you rather than against you. That same flexibility applies to many things, including how your brain deals with **dopamine** levels.

Dopamine is like your internal reward system's fuel. When you experience something enjoyable, your brain pumps out a bit of dopamine, urging you to keep doing that thing. But what happens when there's a shift in this process? Maybe you start leaning into bad habits like scrolling through social media all day or binge-watching TV shows—things that give quick hits of dopamine but offer little long-term satisfaction. Your brain can actually adapt to these habits, relying on that instant dopamine hit more than it should. Neuroplasticity is the reason why this happens, and it's also the way out. Your brain can rewire itself to handle dopamine in a healthier way, but like any change, it takes some work. And a bit of patience.

Now, let's say you want to guide your brain back to a better path—one where dopamine isn't running you into a cycle of short-lived highs and longer lows. You can essentially **train** your brain—sort of like teaching it another new trick. It has the ability to shift gears by forming new connections, making dopamine regulation smoother and more balanced. This could mean learning to enjoy things that offer slower, more enduring rewards, like exercising regularly or picking up a hobby that slowly turns satisfying with practice. The important thing is, whatever route you choose, you're not stuck. Your brain always has the potential to reshape its internal wiring and adjust accordingly. That's what's kind of amazing about neuroplasticity—you're never really locked into one way of thinking or feeling.

As you start making small changes, your brain will kinda follow along. But, it helps to know what **activities** actively help you along this road to better dopamine regulation. So, let's get into some simple, useful exercises that promote this rewiring process—ones that help build a more balanced relationship with dopamine. Here's a list of Neuroplasticity-Enhancing Activities:

• **Physical Exercise**: Jogging, swimming, yoga—whatever gets you moving. Movement leads to more growth factors in the brain. It literally feeds your neurons and keeps them lively.

• Mindfulness **Meditation**: Teaching your brain to stay present instead of trailing off to countless other things. Staying focused in the now trains your brain to treat rewards in a more measured way.

• New Skills or Hobbies: Picking up a musical instrument, committing to learning a foreign language, or tackling any skill that's new to you can flex those brain muscles in ways that slow dopamine down but stretch its effects out.

• Social Connections: Spending quality time with friends or family builds long-term well-being, helping dopamine flow in a healthier manner. Relationships that bring joy without needing constant dopamine hits.

• Getting Enough **Sleep**: Genetics might keep you shorter on sleep some nights, but consistently aiming for rest is crucial—sleep actually helps solidify new neural pathways.

As you practice these activities, the rewiring process won't happen overnight, but your brain will slowly shift to create stronger, more sustainable connections over time. Your **journey** toward healthy dopamine regulation isn't a sprint; it's more of a slow jog, and that's ok. Your brain is flexible, but it works best when given the right tools to gradually tailor itself to new routines.

The Role of Neurotransmitters in Balance

Let's chat about how **brain** chemicals get along. Imagine **dopamine** at the heart of it all—not running the show solo, but working together with others like serotonin and norepinephrine. These chemicals have this crazy intricate relationship, a bit like buddies at a party who've known each other forever. Picture dopamine as the one who gets everyone hyped up, energizing the crowd. But here's the thing: energy needs to be balanced out. That's where serotonin softly steps in. While dopamine's buzzing around spreading **motivation** and excitement, serotonin brings a chill vibe to the mix, promoting feelings of happiness and contentment. It's that calm you feel after nailing something important. It doesn't stop there, though. Norepinephrine's the one in the background, keeping you alert and focused. These three make up a pretty dynamic trio, and their interactions are key to helping you feel motivated, satisfied, and ready to take on whatever's next.

When dopamine's left unchecked, things can get, well, out of hand. Think of your brain like it's hosting this ongoing party, where too much dopamine starts people dancing on the tables—at first, everyone's loving the energy, but keeping that pace up isn't realistic. You'd get burnt out, right? That's why having a balanced serotonin level really matters. When everything's in harmony, serotonin's like signaling for everyone to have a seat, relax, and take some time to feel good about things. That sudden urge to buy something just to feel better? A jolt of dopamine-driven excitement needs calming before it persuades you to make that purchase. This smooth balance of energy and contentment is only possible if you have all these chemicals kept in check—jumping from motivated to relaxed effortlessly, according to what life throws at you.

Let's weave in norepinephrine now and talk about how it ties the loop. You'd see that without it in the picture, the dynamic between dopamine and serotonin might keep clashing against each other.

While dopamine's job is to explore, and serotonin's is to savor those rewards, norepinephrine swoops in ensuring you don't stray too far—keeping focused and stopping you from spiraling into distraction. Like caffeine's effect without making your heart race—raising attention at just the right bits when you're about to lose track. Norepinephrine helps you respond wisely—sticking to goals, assessing risks, knowing when to push a little further, or touching the brakes.

Everything ties into a balanced **system**, which frankly, wouldn't be the powerhouse that it is unless all these chemicals supported one another. Imagine it like each chemical system becomes part of this larger mechanism that's continuously adjusting. The balance isn't just about feeling good; it's about functioning effectively over time. If things tilt too far one way or another, whether dopamine dominates the entire space or norepinephrine pulls you into rigid fixations, harsh imbalances start rolling in toward **mental** health. Feeling like things spin out of control often boils down to demands on one neurochemical outstretching challenges set for the others. You want so many moving parts to fall into step, where chemistry behaves close to an orchestra rather than jumbled instruments all striking out on different tempos.

But let's make it visual—a sort of "Neurotransmitter Balance Wheel" brings all that we've discussed into one complete diagram. Imagine a wheel divided up where each neurochemical takes its portion of this charm, pulled together in ways that complement, nurture, and when behaving rightly, release precisely what you need when you need it. Whether it's a shift toward pursuit, **happiness**, or crisp decision-making, such balancing acts underline that these relationships between dopamine, serotonin, and norepinephrine are less combative and instead supportive allies in creating integration over **emotional** systems.

That wheel spins to project what's working behind daily rhythms you hardly notice: rising in a motivating rush first thing in the morning via dopamine or leaning into your couch after dinner flushed serenely in serotonin's warm glow as you unwind against the subdued "hum" of norepinephrine's quieter focus, reinforcing a healthy flow amidst ever-whirling human experience. Isn't how your brain balances itself out using **neurotransmitters** like an organismic juggling act, just something you'd naturally appreciate a whole lot better knowing what's at play?

Dopamine Receptors and Sensitivity

Let's dive into how those mighty little proteins—**dopamine receptors**—do their thing. These guys are like the gatekeepers for your dopamine signals. When dopamine, that feel-good chemical, gets released in your brain, it needs somewhere to stick, right? That's where receptors come in. They're like docking stations. When dopamine attaches to them, it kick-starts a series of tiny signals that spread through your brain, influencing your mood, motivation, and energy levels.

Here's the tricky part: these receptors aren't always working at full blast. Like most things in your body, their activity isn't constant. If you're constantly flooding your system with dopamine—through things like binge-watching shows, eating lots of sugar, or beating that latest video game—your receptors start adapting. They'll either become less **sensitive** or even reduce in number. Imagine it like this: if you eat too much spicy food, you kind of get used to it, and you need to add more chili just to get that same kick. That's the same deal with dopamine receptors. They start needing more and more to give you the same feeling.

So, what can change these receptors—how sensitive and how many of them there are? This is where the plot thickens. **Genetics** spices things up—certain genes determine how susceptible you are to changes in receptor levels. If your parents had a particular kind of receptor sensitivity, there's a chance that the same thing could happen to you. It's like getting a family hand-me-down, which, in this case, is less about cool furniture and more about how you'd lob dopamine around your neurons.

And it's not just about mom and dad's genes—it's also about your **environment**. The noise around you can mess with your dopamine too. Stress amps up dopamine in the short term but fries your receptors in the long term, making them tired and worn out. The same goes for constant exposure to highly stimulating activities— your environments literally mold your brain by reshaping dopamine behavior. And, boy, the combo of genetics and environment? That can lead to massive swings in mood and motivation.

Alright, so if you've got this mix of genetics, environment, and life choices syncing up, what can you do when you feel your dopamine system is whacked? Allow me to introduce the **Dopamine Receptor Reset Protocol**. This catchy name's more about rebooting your brain tech, just like pressing the reset button on that old Nintendo to get things working from level one again.

Here's how you do it:

• Take a Dopamine Fast: Disconnect. Seriously. Cut your smartphone time, gaming, Netflix binges—anything that's a dopamine bomb—totally out for a day or two. It seems simple, but by getting away from those hits of instant pleasure, you give your neurons time to chill out. Like taking a breather during a tough marathon.

• Get Moving: **Exercise** is a weird one here. It releases dopamine, but it also boosts receptor sensitivity in the long term, making them ready and alert.

• Sleep Well: No-brainer here. Less sleep, messed-up dopamine.

• Mind What You Eat: Your receptors love omega-3 fatty acids, which come loaded in fatty fish like salmon or supplements. Also, don't neglect antioxidants—they sort of protect your receptors.

• Try **Meditation**: When you're mindful, your baseline dopamine levels tend to recalibrate to healthier levels.

And here's some truth—it's not all done in a week or two. This is a reset—it's about laying good foundations. But when your dopamine receptors are more sensitive and responsive, life's little pleasures, well, they feel a whole lot bigger.

So, taking the time to treat your **dopaminergic system** just right? It might just refill the joy tank and get you all jacked up for life and your goals... without needing that extra spicy hit every time.

The Dopamine-Stress Connection

Alright, let's talk about how **stress** throws your **dopamine** outta whack. Ever noticed how when you're stressed, it's like your **motivation** and **mood** just go down the drain? Well, that's no coincidence. Stress, dopamine, and cortisol are constantly in this tricky dance. When you're in a stressful situation, your body pumps out cortisol—which is like your "Uh-oh, things are getting bad!" alert system. Normally, there's nothing wrong with a little bit of stress. But when it sticks around for too long? That's when you start running into problems.

Now, how does this relate to dopamine? Think of dopamine as the thing that keeps you going, like a car's **engine**. It's what buzzes in your brain when you accomplish stuff, making you feel good. But cortisol—the stress hormone—tends to mess with it. When you're all stressed out, cortisol sort of hogs your brain's attention, which means dopamine isn't really getting the spotlight it needs. Over time, this can result in issues like feeling unmotivated or even slipping into depression. In short, stress doesn't just make you feel bad in the moment—it can mess up how your brain works in the long run, too.

You might notice that you're not as happy or driven as you used to be. That's stress messing with your dopamine signals, making them less effective. It's like someone is lowering the volume on your feel-good music, and suddenly everything sounds dull. You're chasing that same excitement or joy from before, but it's just not there because stressed-out dopamine doesn't work as it should. The more stress you pile on, the worse it gets—like a snowball gathering speed down the hill. Pretty soon, you're stuck in a bad cycle.

So, what can you do? You've gotta find a way to keep that cortisol in check. And that's where we introduce the "Stress-Dopamine **Regulation** Technique." Fancy title—simple idea. It's all about small actions you can take when stress starts creeping in so you don't wreck your dopamine balance. You're not gonna be swamped, just tiny adjustments to help your brain stay on-track.

First up: Identify when you're stressed out. Get used to noticing how you're feeling mentally and physically. Are your shoulders tight? Is your heart beating fast? Maybe you're tense, not laughing like usual, or just down for no reason. That's when you've got to pause. Take a deep **breath**, like in and out slow, then refocus. Meditation or mindfulness might help, but if that's not your jam, try simple activities you enjoy—something like playing your favorite song or going for a quick walk. These little things let your brain relax so it doesn't drown in cortisol.

Next is planning breaks. It's really easy to just push through stressful situations. But taking a short break where you unplug can be magic for reset. During these breaks, you give your brain a moment to recover, and bam—dopamine levels can come up for air. It's quick, it's not complicated, and it's keeping that balance in check.

Last, keep things around you that make you laugh or smile. Sounds tiny, right? But these small bits of joy matter. Adding some lightness daily keeps dopamine flowing in a good direction. Tiny boosts that counterbalance stress—while proving to your brain and your body that everything is going to be okay.

So, that's the scoop: Stress messes with your dopamine system in a real way, but there are steps—small, easy steps—that can stop that spiral. By fitting the "Stress-Dopamine Regulation Technique" into your routine, you hang on to your **motivation** and good vibes, even when stress lurks around the corner. Sure—it might take some practice, but you're making space for your brain to bounce back stronger and more balanced next time stress decides to drop in unannounced.

In Conclusion

In this chapter, you've taken a deeper dive into how the **brain** can change and adapt when it comes to **dopamine**. You've seen how dopamine isn't just a single entity working solo; it's interconnected with other brain chemicals, and these connections can influence how you feel, think, and act daily. These concepts aren't just theoretical—they can be practically applied to boost your **well-being**.

You've learned about how **neuroplasticity** allows your brain to rewire itself and change based on your habits and environment. You've discovered why dopamine works closely with other brain chemicals like serotonin and norepinephrine—all of which need to collaborate for a balanced mind. You've also seen that you can purposefully choose activities to keep your brain's dopamine regulation on track.

The importance of dopamine **receptors** in the brain has been highlighted, along with how their sensitivity can change based on various factors. You've explored the connection between **stress** and dopamine, understanding how excessive stress can disrupt your dopamine levels, leading to imbalance.

Now, it's time to put what you've learned into **practice**, keeping your brain robust and balanced. These methods can help you feel better today and maintain a steady mind for the long haul. Remember, the goal is to create a **lifestyle** that supports healthy dopamine function, which in turn supports your overall mental well-being.

So, mate, why not start implementing some of these ideas? Your brain will thank you for it, and you might just find yourself feeling more balanced and energized as a result. It's all about making small, consistent changes that add up to big improvements in your mental health over time.

Chapter 6: Nutrition for Dopamine Balance

Ever felt like life is a **balancing** act, and your mood is the tightrope? Trust me, I've been there. We all know how important it is to feel **motivated** and focused, but the secret sauce that makes everything click is **dopamine**. And guess what? It doesn't just happen—you're actually in **control**. No, it's not magic. It's about what you put in your body, and that's exactly what this chapter digs into.

So why is it that some days you're on **fire**, while other times, you can't even think straight? Well, let's dive into what you **eat**, drink, and even when you do it. Imagine having the power to design your **meals** in a way that boosts your dopamine and your **mood** altogether.

Get ready to take the reins. You're not just eating; you're fueling your brain and body for success. By making smart choices about your nutrition, you can actually influence how you feel and perform throughout the day. It's like being the DJ of your own mental soundtrack—you get to choose the tunes that keep you grooving.

This chapter is your backstage pass to understanding how food affects your dopamine levels. You'll learn which foods can give you that natural high and which ones might be throwing a wrench in your mental gears. It's not about strict diets or cutting out everything you love. It's about making informed choices that help you feel your best.

So, buckle up, buddy. You're about to embark on a tasty journey that could change the way you think about food—and yourself. Ready to fuel up and feel awesome? Let's dive in!

Foods That Naturally Enhance Dopamine

Ever wonder how your **diet** could mess with or, even better, help your **mood**? Let's talk about foods that can naturally bump up your dopamine levels. Dopamine's like the brain's "feel-good" chemical, right? It keeps your **motivation** engine running smoothly and gives you that little spark to get stuff done. But like any good engine, it needs the right fuel. This is where food comes in.

If we're talking about dopamine, we've got to start with the building blocks. Think of dopamine as a Lego creation. Tyrosine and phenylalanine are the little pieces that make it up. Without enough of these, your brain can't make that feel-good dopamine. And where do these pieces come from? You've got it—your diet. Foods like eggs, dairy, chicken, fish, and turkey are packed with the stuff. Another one is soy products like tofu—great for the non-meat eaters out there.

You also won't want to skip out on seeds, nuts, and some beans, like lentils and chickpeas. All chock-full of the ammo your body needs. Don't forget, fruits like bananas bring a solid dose too. Nuts like almonds and walnuts are classics, a perfect handful for a quick boost. Not the kind that makes you jittery, just that good steady feeling like you're on top of things. A little reminder to treat your **brain** like the VIP it is.

You're probably thinking, why does it matter? Can't you just eat whatever as long as you take vitamins or something? Fair question. But balance isn't something you can just pill your way into. Your brain needs a consistent supply of what's real and wholesome. Like a vehicle that runs better on premium rather than unleaded. Tyrosine-rich stuff does more than give you a dopamine nudge. Over time, it supports you when you need to stay focused or give that project your all.

Moving on. Tyrosine and phenylalanine don't do their job alone, and this is where certain **nutrients** cozy in. You need folks like B6, iron, folate, and a mix of other vitamins to really get dopamine moving from assembly to the "feel-good party" in your brain. They make tyrosine do its thing by ensuring enzymes work right, processes keep up, you know all the functions that keep the brain clicking.

Leafy veggies like spinach give you that much-needed folate. Beef and turkey match up for that B6 and iron. It's teamwork in action here, all part of keeping that motivation wheel turning while saying goodbye to just functioning on fumes.

Now, let's have some fun—and by fun, I mean cooking. **Food** can become your best ally in this dopamine game, with a mix of stuff that's easy and gets you these brain goodies all at once. Hence, welcome the "Dopamine-Boosting Recipe Collection." Think meals like a turkey kale salad with some almond zest. Super simple, right? Or maybe do scrambled eggs with spinach and a sprinkle of cheese. It's got the whole combo for that brain jolt you're after.

Or try roasted chickpeas with some lemon and garlic—those babies fall into that tasty and nutritious sweet spot. For dessert lovers, a banana walnut smoothie could be your new morning go-to. Smash bananas with walnuts, add almond milk, maybe throw some dates in there if you like a sweet touch. Great way to start your day, really.

Bringing tasty into **healthy eating** is possible, easier than you'd think and much more satisfying in the long run. Your brain will thank you for the little tweaks with more clarity, better mood, and less roller-coaster emotions. Whole natural foods, cooked into something your mind and body enjoy, truly do play a huge part in how peppy or sluggish you feel that day.

Supplements and Their Effect on Dopamine

Have you ever gazed into your pantry, wondering if there were magic pills to make your brain feel better? Well, here's the scoop: kinda. Several supplements out there target **dopamine**, your brain's feel-good chemical. Some work like a charm in the right conditions, but there are always trade-offs, right? Balancing dopamine isn't just a "pop a pill and you're done" kind of deal.

When it comes to supplements that influence dopamine, a few stand out like reliable old buddies—you know, the ones who actually show up on time. **L-tyrosine** is one of them. It's an amino acid you also get from food (like chicken or turkey), but in supplement form, it can ramp up dopamine production for some folks. It's like revving up your engine after it's been slacking off. The idea is simple: give your brain more of the building blocks it needs to make dopamine and see if it swings things in your favor.

Then there's **Mucuna Pruriens**—fancy name, but it's basically a bean that's been around in Ayurvedic practices forever. This "dopamine bean" naturally contains L-DOPA, the same stuff doctors prescribe for people with Parkinson's disease. It's potent, giving your brain exactly what it needs to crank out dopamine like it's a limited-edition sneaker drop. Sure, it can help you feel more motivated or perhaps balance out that brain fog, but don't let that fool you—it's a strong brew, and you probably want to approach it with a bit of respect.

Rhodiola Rosea is another brain-friendly supplement that's come across our radar. Unlike the direct-building stuff like L-tyrosine and Mucuna Pruriens, Rhodiola takes a broader approach. It's an adaptogen, which means it vibes with your overall stress levels and supports mental function by balancing out cortisol (your stress hormone), indirectly affecting dopamine. It's like setting the mood lighting for your brain to chill out and work better all at the same time.

Now, before you race to stock up your supplement cabinet, let's think about the fine print. Sure, these could make your brain feel a bit more "you," but overdoing it isn't a great plan. Too much dopamine stimulation could backfire, like one of those fireworks you set off a bit too low to the ground. You overshoot it, and you might start dealing with anxiety, through-the-roof energy, or even aggression.

There's also the fact that not all supplements mix well. If you overdose on dopamine supplements together, it's kind of like mixing too many strong cocktails: it can result in a bad time, no doubt. L-tyrosine might get your brain pumping dopamine, but if you're loading it up with a high dose of Mucuna Pruriens too, you could end up in overdrive. Plus, there's always the factor of quality; not all supplement brands are created equal, and not every pill in the bottle's gonna be top shelf.

Alright, it isn't all doom-and-gloom. There's actually a way to make this safer and way more effective—something I'd call a "consideration guide." Let's look at what I'd label as a **"Dopamine Support Supplement Stack."** Here's a simple approach:

• Start with L-tyrosine: A moderate dose in the morning boosts your brain with the basic tools it needs. No more, no less. Sort of like sharpening your pencil before you need to write.

• Add in Rhodiola Rosea if you're dealing with a stressful day: This could help regulate stress which messes with dopamine production. It helps keep your brain on an even keel, nothing too crazy.

• Reserve Mucuna Pruriens for when you really need a dopamine jolt: Maybe you've got a tough project or a bunch of things to get through—this gives you a strong lift, but use it sparingly to avoid getting into overstimulation mode.

This 'stack' makes it easier to play it smart and not blow things out of proportion, which pretty much sums up what we're after, isn't it? When used carefully—and smart—these **supplements** can give your brain a bit of an assist without the wild side effects.

Transitioning from dealing with what supplements often promise, those gains can quickly run off the cliff of overdoing things. It's all about **balance**, really. Keep that in mind, and you'll be on your way to a more balanced, dopamine-friendly lifestyle.

The Importance of Hydration in Dopamine Production

Ever feel like your **brain's** running on empty, as if no matter what you do, you're dragging through the day? Well, your water intake might be playing a bigger role than you realize. Staying properly **hydrated** isn't just about avoiding dehydration; it's central to how your brain functions—including how it produces key chemicals like **dopamine**, which is basically the "feel-good" messenger in your noggin.

Dopamine isn't just some abstract idea; it's what makes you feel **motivated**, enjoy certain activities, and stay focused. When you're well-hydrated, your brain cells have what they need to keep the dopamine flowing. Water helps ensure that nutrients are transported effectively, and toxins are removed. It's like keeping a garden well-watered so everything can grow right. If your brain were that garden, then dopamine would be the plants soaking up all the stuff they need to bloom. But what happens if you stop watering that garden? Spoiler: It's not pretty.

Let's say you skimp on **water**. Maybe it's just 'cause you're busy, or you forget to drink enough during the day. A lack of hydration slows everything down. Those plants we mentioned? Well, they're going to wilt. With less dopamine, your brain struggles to do its job. Your mood tanks, you feel unmotivated, and unless you drink some water soon, **productivity** basically goes out the window. You become sluggish, irritable, and straight-up foggy in the head; it's hard to concentrate on anything. Funny enough, just when you need that dopamine the most, your brain's too dehydrated to make enough of it.

So, what's the fix? It's pretty straightforward—just drink more water. But like most things in life, it's easier said than done. The trick is to make hydration an ongoing **habit**, instead of a reactive measure when you start feeling low.

Here are some of the best hydration tips to make sure your brain stays dopamine-happy:

• Always Have a Water Bottle Handy: And fill it up throughout the day. Sip on it, don't gulp. You're more likely to drink regularly when it's within reach.

• Eat Water-Rich Foods: Fruits like watermelon, cucumbers, and oranges aren't just tasty—they also provide a good chunk of your daily water intake without you even realizing it. Kind of like sneaking revision into something you're already doing.

• Set Timer Reminders: Your phone isn't just there for texts and social feeds—it can remind you to get that H2O in regularly. Set a timer every hour or so to drink a glass.

• Pay Attention to Your Pee: Yeah, you read that right. The clearer it is, the better hydrated you are. If it's turning dark yellow, that's your body screaming for some hydration help.

As you stay properly hydrated, that foggy feeling will lift, and along with it, your brain's ability to produce dopamine at healthy levels. You'll be more motivated, your mood will be more balanced, and your thinking will clear up in no time. So, while it sounds ridiculously simple, drinking enough water consistently is something you can't afford to overlook. Think of it as a basic foundation—a well-watered garden where everything else thrives.

Meal Timing and Dopamine Levels

You might think of **dopamine** as something your brain pumps out after a big win or when you've conquered a challenge. But it's not just about those major moments. Surprisingly, the **timing** of your meals plays a huge role in how well your dopamine functions daily. Pretty interesting, right?

Here's the deal: Your brain reactively releases dopamine based on regular routines like eating. When you eat at the same times each day, you're basically training your brain to release dopamine on that schedule. Just like that, lunchtime or dinnertime might become one of those **anticipated** moments simply because your brain's gotten used to the rhythm.

The tricky part comes when you don't stick to a schedule. Imagine skipping meals or overeating randomly. That irregularity messes with consistent dopamine release. Instead of having stable dopamine flowing throughout the day, it uses up your brain's dopamine store inefficiently — leaving you craving more frequent hits. This can lead to choosing unhealthy snacks to spike your dopamine or having lots of moments feeling off.

But get this: **fasting** every so often could actually bring a brighter, sharper tune to your dopamine system. And when I say "fasting," I don't mean starving yourself. It's all about intermittent fasting. You'd be setting specific windows for your meals instead of eating throughout the day. There's something cool about it. By reducing your eating window, you might just increase that dopamine sensitivity. You know that saying, less is more? This approach trades the cost of constantly searching for that next snack or digital distraction with intervals where your brain learns to become more responsive.

With intermittent fasting (or even just setting smaller eating windows than you currently do), your brain learns to release dopamine more efficiently during those times you do eat. There's a sense of higher **satisfaction** from your meals — and it's not messed up by late-night snacks or leftover feelings of hunger. Because when you stop overloading your dopamine stores, your brain opens up with a better, more honest response. Each meal feels more fulfilling, and your overall daily mood becomes more regular and stable.

Here's how to think about it for yourself. Start figuring out times when your meals really hit the spot — respond to that by finding a rhythm and sticking to it. Develop what I like to call a "Dopamine-Optimized Meal Schedule." It's a simple plan:

• Set your daily eating window: Begin and end eating within an 8-10 hour period.

• Have your meals during consistent hours: Breakfast is always within the same hour after the eating window starts. Lunch should be square in the middle. The last meal is no closer than two hours before your window closes.

• Make space for fasting: During non-eating hours, steer yourself away from looking for quick fixes with an extra snack or candy.

• Strengthen your mental habit: Align mental tasks with this meal schedule. Like working on important goals or engaging in creative hobbies right after lunch, making use of your afternoon pump in dopamine.

This plan might sound strict at first, especially if you're used to grazing. But with some steady practice, it helps lower those wild fluctuations and creates a thriving dopamine rhythm. The result? Rewarding **clarity** and sustained **motivation** throughout the day.

So, meal timing goes hand in hand with everything you're trying to achieve: a more balanced and predictable sense of well-being, better focus, and above all, feeling good day-to-day without overworking your brain's dopamine system. Why not give it some thought? You might find it changes the way you experience food and mood alike.

Practical Exercise: Designing a Dopamine-Friendly Meal Plan

Alright, you've **decided** to improve your diet to give your dopamine levels some love. Awesome! But before you start adding cool new foods to your grocery list or creating a Pinterest-worthy meal plan, there's something crucial you need to do first: take a hard look at what you're already eating. Yeah, I know—looking back can sometimes be a bit of a buzzkill. Maybe you've found yourself glued to the couch, mindlessly munching on snacks that probably aren't helping you feel any sharper or more motivated. It's all good, though. **Awareness** is the first step, right? Jot down what you typically eat in a week. Breakfast weirdly inconsistent? Relying a little too much on takeout? Dig deep and note it all down. You're not here to judge yourself; you're here to improve. It's about honing in on the little habits you don't think much about but are making all the difference.

When you've got that list in front of you, think about where you're able to make upgrades. Not massive overhauls, but changes here and there. Maybe it's swapping out that sugary cereal in the morning with something heartier—like oatmeal with nuts and berries. Or adding a few more greens to your dinner plate versus that extra helping of fries. You're looking for areas where you can gently nudge things toward being dopamine-friendly.

Got those ideas? Great! Because you'll need them as we step into phase two of the plan—making a list of foods that can actually help bump up your dopamine. You're probably wondering, which foods do that exactly? Well, the magic mostly happens with foods rich in amino acids, particularly **tyrosine**—because tyrosine is like the raw material your brain uses to create dopamine. Consider adding things like turkey, chicken, eggs, beans, and fish. Next, think about including more omega-3-rich foods like salmon or walnuts, because omega-3s help keep your brain firing on all cylinders. Oh, and don't overlook the power of dark leafy greens—they're loaded with vitamins and minerals that not only feed your body but also fuel your brain.

With your list in hand, it's now time to start sketching out what an entire dopamine-friendly week looks like. Think Sunday-to-Saturday, but with fewer processed snacks and maybe a bit more of those tyrosine-boosting foods. It's super important to strike a **balance** here. If you're prone to steering clear of breakfast, ease yourself in. Think smoothies loaded with berries and seeds or a good egg-hash combo. And don't shy away from repetition— it's actually easier to stick with, and nobody will judge you for having yogurt parfait two days in a row. Before you know it, you'll have a road map for the next week that keeps you full and fuels that dopamine wave you've been craving.

But food timing can mess with your groove. You know how you can feel sluggish when you eat a meal at a weird time? Sorting out when to eat can seriously level up how you feel. Eating that late-night snack? Probably not doing you favors. Some folks move their meals earlier, while others swear by **intermittent fasting**. You eat deliberately in a shorter window—maybe between noon and 8 PM—and skip breakfast. Fast in the morning, that is, not the whole day. This shorter eating window can kick off higher dopamine production and prevent those sluggish dips in energy.

With all the set pieces in play, it's time to **execute**. Go through with the plan for a week and keep tabs on how you're doing. Carry a notepad if you need to, or use a phone app. Were you energized after that protein-packed lunch or a little irritable because you forgot your mid-afternoon snack? Whatever happens, log those changes—notice where you felt a difference in mood or motivation. Food is fuel, and seeing the health benefits in real-time can reinforce that.

After you've stuck to that for a bit, think about making **tweaks**—you might realize that afternoon snack was key for not going on a chocolate bender later in the evening or that fasting doesn't sit well with you. We're all wired a bit differently, so it's cool to shuffle things around until you find what works.

Finally, as you start noticing what works for your dopamine, lean more into it. Gradually add these good eating habits across all meals. A little cocoa here, more fish there. New meals might even inspire you to try more. By easing all this into action, you're setting the intentional slow and steady rhythm for genuine **change**. Way to go! You're creating a fresher, better platform for both your body and brain. Keep the momentum up, day in and day out, by consistently upgrading what you put on your plate.

In Conclusion

This chapter shines a spotlight on the **vital role** nutrition plays in supporting and balancing **dopamine levels** in your body, ultimately affecting your mood, motivation, and overall well-being. Through detailed explanations and practical tips, you're now equipped with the knowledge you need to make conscious **dietary choices** that naturally enhance dopamine.

In this chapter, you've discovered:

• How certain foods rich in tyrosine and phenylalanine can help **boost dopamine** levels in your brain.

• The benefit of specific nutrients like magnesium, B-vitamins, and omega-3 fats in supporting healthy dopamine function.

• A **recipe collection** designed to incorporate dopamine-boosting ingredients into tasty everyday meals.

• Safe and effective **supplements** that contribute positively to dopamine balance, along with their potential risks.

• The impact of meal timing, particularly **intermittent fasting**, on enhancing the synchronization of dopamine release with your body's natural rhythms.

As you move forward, consider incorporating the best practices from this chapter into your daily life to foster a balanced and sustainable approach to **dopamine production**. Small, consistent changes to your diet can have a powerful effect on your mood and motivation, enabling you to take full advantage of your body's natural chemistry. Always remember that the power to positively influence your mental and emotional health starts with the choices you make on your plate.

Chapter 7: Physical Activity and Dopamine

Ever felt like there was a secret **switch** in your brain that, if flipped, could make you feel unstoppable? You've probably been there too—wondering what it takes to get through the day with **energy** and focus. That's what we're diving into in this chapter. And no, it's not some magic pill or complicated process; it's something you can do every day. In fact, you might already be doing it, but probably aren't aware of its true **power**.

You're about to discover how simple **movements**—maybe ones you've not even thought much about—can totally transform how you feel. I'll show you how different types of **activity** can turn that switch on and how to find the sweet spot between effort and pleasure. Ready to see just how much you can change your everyday life with this? You'll even work on putting together a **plan** that fits perfectly into your routine.

Get ready to unlock the secrets of physical activity and its impact on your brain's **dopamine** levels. You'll learn how to harness this natural **high** to boost your mood, increase your productivity, and enhance your overall well-being. From quick desk exercises to more intense workouts, you'll find options that suit your lifestyle and preferences.

So, are you excited to transform your daily grind into an opportunity for growth and vitality? Let's jump right in and explore how you can leverage physical activity to become the best version of yourself.

Exercise as a Natural Dopamine Enhancer

Whenever you throw on those sneakers and hit the pavement or gym, there's something happening inside your **brain** that might surprise you. It's like flipping a switch and turning your own dopamine faucet on. That **neurotransmitter** responsible for your motivation, connection, and I'd even say – happiness. When you start to move, your neurons have a party, releasing more dopamine right away. And on top of all that, your brain starts to get better at recognizing and using this dopamine. Exercise is like training your brain to enjoy the hits of dopamine it gets—helping it get more out of every drop. Pretty nifty, right?

Right off the bat, while you're working those **muscles** and getting a sweat on, dopamine starts to do its thing. Ever notice how after a good **workout** you feel almost giddy, totally energized, or just ready to tackle what's next? That's your dopamine kicking it into high gear. It rushes to your brain, taking your mood up a notch and making you feel strong, positive, and, well, pretty accomplished. Even after you hit the showers, that feel-good rush sticks around, calming you down and chilling you out in the best way.

But here's the cool thing about working out – it doesn't just change your mood for now. Stick with an exercise routine for a while – a few months, let's say – and something amazing starts to happen. Your brain becomes more sensitive to that dopamine, making those good vibes easier to catch. You're not just chasing a temporary high, you're actually training your brain to become a steady dopamine machine. Like conditioning your muscles, you're conditioning that grey matter to respond better over time. So not only do your workouts boost **mood** and **motivation** today, but they also set you up to feel better, more focused, and motivated in everything else you go after. It's kinda like planting seeds today and enjoying the harvest later.

So how do you cash in on this? Easy! By weaving **exercise** into your life in a way that keeps these dopamine taps flowing over time. It's not about hitting the gym for hours every day or training like an athlete. All you really need is the right type of workouts sprinkled into your week to keep that brain pumpin' happily.

To boost your dopamine through workouts, try mixing up your routine:

• Focus on aerobic stuff – something that gets your blood going and your heart rate up. Think brisk walks, jogs, biking, or even just dancing like nobody's watching. These bouts of movement trigger that dopamine surge. Aim for about 30 minutes at least three to five times a week.

• Don't forget strength workouts – lifting weights at the gym, bodyweight exercises at home, or even yoga. There's something about building muscle and challenging your body that gives your brain a kick, too.

• Make time for stretching – calming your body down after a workout can help you relax and reset that dopamine balance.

• End with something playful – fun workouts like swimming, biking with buddies, or even something silly like obstacle course races that spike your dopamine while having a good time. It's like tricking yourself into being healthy.

Together, these types of exercises not only get your body into shape but keep those dopamine levels balanced. The more you make these routines a **habit**, the more steadily you'll feed your brain with what it craves – stable motivation, clearer thinking, better moods, and oh... just feeling dang good about yourself.

The Effect of Various Exercise Types

Ever wonder why some workouts leave you **buzzing** with energy and others just make you feel tired? It's all about how different exercises tap into your body's **dopamine** system—yup, the same system that gets triggered by your favorite guilty pleasure, but way healthier! Cardio, like running or cycling, gives you a steady release of dopamine, filling you with that "runner's high." It's like a slow drip of happiness that sustains over time, keeping you motivated and on the go. If you're cooler with a jog on a Sunday morning, this one's your jam.

On the other hand, if you're a fan of **weightlifting**, you already know it's a different kind of rush. Every time you go for that heavy lift and feel the strain, your body pumps out a powerful burst of dopamine. It's not just the grind—it's the thrill of challenging your limits that cranks up those dopamine levels. Pushing through tough reps can leave you feeling like you just conquered a mountain, even if you've never stepped foot outside the gym.

So, cardio equals sustained happiness, while weightlifting is that quick shot of joy and **excitement**—two very different but equally awesome ways to get that dopamine flowing. Gotta say, it sounds like having both is just the right recipe for keeping things energized and satisfying.

But here's where it gets even more interesting! Trying out new **exercises** or shaking things up with tougher routines can actually supercharge your dopamine hit. Imagine trying something new, like taking up boxing or going for a spin class when you've done nothing but treadmill running forever. The more your brain realizes it's facing something unfamiliar and challenging, the more dopamine it hands out, like a "job well done!" sticker. And that buzz you feel during and after the workout? It's the result of your brain celebrating those new stimuli.

It's sort of like learning to play a game for the first time. At first, it's the novelty that pumps you up. You're extra focused, fully immersed in the action. Each new punch, spin, or squat awakens a part of you since this is out of your regular routine. And what happens? Your brain caters to you with a higher dopamine kick for your bravery in stepping outside your usual comfort zone. The pleasure keeps rolling in, almost as if your mind is trying to coax you into making a habit out of this new, challenging experience.

To keep this adrenaline high on regular, you'll need an assortment of different workouts. Enter the "Exercise **Variety** Matrix"—your go-to for mixing up those workouts just right! The matrix works by balancing cardio, strength training, and those fun, challenging exercises you may have shied away from before. Start with your steady playlist of activities—like running on Monday, maybe some strength training on Wednesday, then add a new one come Friday, like yoga or rock climbing.

The goal here is variety because variety is basically fear's worst enemy and pleasure's best friend. Switching things up forces your brain to adapt, which boosts your dopamine production in unexpected ways. Keep a conscious effort to mix workouts. Leg days with ab days, running with skipping—play around! Your body will start to anticipate something new, keeping that rewarding dopamine hit around longer.

Consistency? It's like unlocking the secret sauce of feeling that dopamine high as often as you lace up your sneakers or grip that barbell. Plus, by building a good mix, you don't just train your body but your mind too. All while keeping your brain happy on the dopamine train.

And that, right there, could be your secret to catching that sometimes-elusive balance and a dash of zest in how you move each day. Different workouts, different kinds of **satisfaction**. All giving you what you need when you need it most.

Optimal Duration and Intensity for Dopamine Release

When you're aiming to keep your **dopamine** levels in check while working out, getting the length and intensity just right is key. You don't have to overdo it; you want that sweet spot where you're maximizing benefits without tipping into burnout territory.

So, what's the perfect **workout** length? Generally, about 30 to 45 minutes per session is the ideal range. This strikes the right balance between keeping your workouts effective without veering into overkill. They should be tough enough to get your heart pumping but not so tough that you're utterly drained after. You know that feeling, where you've pushed just enough to sweat out the stress but not so hard you're wrecked the next day. It's not about running a marathon every time you hit the gym; it's about having a routine that you can maintain. That's how you keep those dopamine levels thriving without risk of overexertion.

Now, a little note on **intensity**. You want to mix in both moderate and intense workouts. If you're the type who enjoys a good run, you might want to vary between a light jog and some sprints. Or if you're into lifting weights, switch up between medium and heavy sets. The exact approach will differ depending on what your body craves, but the main idea is to shoot for that blend of moderate effort and short bursts where you give it your all.

So, pulling that 30 to 45 minutes into view again, do the trick by switching things up—like every other day, play with intensity a bit. Moderate pace one day; more intense fitness fun the next. That way, you're keeping your dopamine stirred up, ready to roll, without overloading it.

But while we're on the topic of keeping things under control, let me throw this out there: a little bit of **stress** from exercise? It's actually good for your dopamine. This might sound kinda weird at first, but here's what it boils down to. You don't want to live in a perpetual state of relaxation—it's boring, and boredom doesn't do anything for dopamine release. What you need is a bit of the 'good' stress that nudges your body to challenge itself. When you feel that muscle burn or when you're out of breath (without feeling like you might pass out), that's your body's way of adapting to stress. And conveniently, it triggers a surge of dopamine, giving you that sense of accomplishment as you push through.

But, set reasonable **expectations**. Just a sprinkle of stress during workouts will keep dopamine afloat. Go too far though, and you'll wear yourself out—hello, fatigue. The problem with running on empty is, instead of boosting your mood, it can do the opposite, leaving you feeling a bit down or "meh." So, hone in on that line—right where you push up against what's challenging, but not punishing.

So, here's a little something that puts it all together—a Dopamine-Optimized Exercise Prescription, if you will. This'll help tailor your workouts for just the right mix of time and intensity, plus a hint of good stress:

• Whether you're lifting weights, running, or shaking it up at a dance class, aim for 30 to 45-minute sessions, at least 4 days a week.

• Alternate between moderate workouts and more intense drill days. On mild days, you're working slightly above a leisurely pace. Intense days? Yeah, you're full throttle, but only in short spurts.

• Ensure that for every hard burst of exercise, there's a cool down—a laid-back period that winds everything down smoothly.

• Keep the 'good stress'—burn in those muscles, sweat on your brow, but back off well before anything starts to feel too uncomfortable.

Stick to something like this, cater it to how you're feeling—and most importantly, keep it **enjoyable**. The trick is to carry forward that sense of pace and progression where your dopamine levels rise without throwing you into extremes. Find that point, and you'll have nailed the sporting **balance** that keeps both body and mind humming along.

Incorporating Movement into Daily Life

We all know how **tricky** it can be fitting exercise into an already packed schedule. But moving around more doesn't always mean you've got to hit the gym. It's more about finding **creative** ways to keep your body active through those regular, everyday activities. And believe me, small tweaks can make a big difference in keeping your **dopamine** in check while you're at it.

So, start with your coffee routine. Instead of grabbing a seat, how about you take a ten-minute **walk** with that cup? Stretch while waiting for the coffee to brew or simply pace up and down while catching up on your messages. It's subtle but it'll wake you up more, and keep those dopamine levels from dipping first thing in the morning.

Next, think about your daily tasks—taking the stairs instead of the elevator, parking a little further from your destination, or standing up whenever you're on the phone. Standing desk setups are great too if you can swap to one. These little habits might seem small but over time they all add up—each one giving you a tiny bit of that extra **movement** throughout the day.

What's cool about incorporating more non-exercise activity throughout your day is that it fights against those long sit-and-stare habits. When you sit for hours on end, your body and your mood get sluggish. That hit of movement, even a little, acts as a trigger— you flip from lazy-mode to alert-mode instantly.

Now, if you're wondering how to keep the **energy** rolling throughout your day, it's like hitting 'refresh.' That's where frequent movement breaks come into play.

When you've been stuck at a desk for way too long, get up! Do a light stretch, walk a lap around the room, step outside for five minutes—anything to get the blood flowing again. You could set a timer to remind you every hour or so. In case you're on the go, even standing and shifting around a bit can make a difference. You've probably noticed how folks are doing "getting steps in" bursts—they get up to stretch their legs during lunch or between breaks—turns out, that's not just a modern habit, it's about keeping those feel-good chemicals steady and your dopamine humming evenly instead of crashing.

And consider the brain as this aging computer that gets 'clogged'—lengthy sitting contributes to that brain fog, but quick breaks, for instance, help the brain hit that reset button. Walking or stretching, even if just for a minute, has this wild way of giving your brain that reboot it needs.

Alright, this brings me to the Dopamine Micro-Movement Plan. It's not as fancy as it might sound—it's all about mini-workouts you can easily sneak in.

Let me assure you, anyone can start this plan without stressing over sore muscles or spending extra time on fitness. Here's the deal: whenever you've got a two-minute window, throw in a micro-movement. It could be 20 jumping jacks, a minute of brisk walking or short stretches. Some options include touching your toes, doing wall squats (just lean and slide down an empty wall), or desk push-ups—yes, the desk you sit at can work wonders during these tiny pockets of time.

This idea is simpler than timing yourself at the gym: sprinkle these little moves all over your job time. Waiting for something to heat in the microwave? Squat for those 30 seconds. Ads showing with streaming? Perfect thirty-second window for toe-touches or lunges. If sitting long hours doesn't kill you, slow movement surely boosts those essentials in your brain, spreading out your **energy** evenly.

And there's something neat about all that—it's free! There's no cost, no equipment. By adding in bits of micro-movements like adding seasoning to food, getting bursts of dopamine gets underlying lazy blocks scraped away, leaving **longevity** behind. Over time, bitty bits add up—an overall shift in bringing you consistent focus, better mood, and without even real exercise. Try it—it doesn't change up your whole day, you just slip it into cracks of free time. Isn't that worth it?

It's where science meets casual life—a fresher balance one move at a time.

Practical Exercise: Creating a Dopamine-Boosting Workout Plan

If you want to tap into the natural feel-good chemicals your brain can produce, it's essential to have a **workout** plan that fits your lifestyle and preferences. The first thing you'll want to consider in creating this plan is your current **fitness** level and what kinds of exercise actually appeal to you. Figuring this out is important because if what you're doing doesn't genuinely interest you, the odds of sticking with the plan are pretty slim. Do you like more intense activities, like running or weightlifting, or do you prefer something a bit slower paced, like yoga or walking? Think about what kinds of exercises you've tried in the past—what left you feeling **energized** and motivated? Got it? You're already on the right track.

Once you've thought about your preferences and fitness level, you can start choosing **activities** that match both what you enjoy and your goals. If your fitness level is low, start small—even a daily 20-minute walk is a great start. On the other hand, if you're more active, you might want to add some variety to keep things interesting. Mix things up with some cardio, like jogging or cycling, paired with resistance exercises such as bodyweight workouts or hitting the gym for weightlifting. Throwing in an enjoyable class—like Zumba, for example—could make things even more effective, keeping you motivated and giving you something to look forward to.

Next, **timing** is something to think about. Identifying the best times for exercise is important because it can really help with that dopamine release. If you want to spike your energy levels for the day, morning workouts are great. You get that dopamine rush to shake off any grogginess and feel alert. On the flip side, if mornings aren't your thing, try late afternoon or early evening, right before the day winds down but before you start your nighttime routine. You can experiment and figure out what clicks for you. Flexibility matters too, so leave room to shift things around based on how you're feeling.

Moving on, make sure to keep your exercise plan varied. Sticking to just one form of exercise might not keep your brain or body fully engaged. In a typical week, mix it up—do some cardio to get your heart pumping and promote a steady release of **dopamine**, some strength training to give those muscles a reason to grow, and add something newer or challenging into the mix. Throw in a class you've never done before, or try that new workout method everyone's talking about—keeping things fresh will give you that little dopamine boost we're aiming for.

While having structured workouts is key, don't neglect those short **movement** breaks. If you spend a lot of time sitting—whether it's at the office, behind a computer, or binge-watching shows—stand up every hour or so. A quick stretch, a couple of squats, or even dancing through a song can recharge you and help maintain that feel-good energy.

To make sure you're creating some sort of positive cycle, take note of how your mood, energy, and **motivation** levels change as you stick with your workout plan. Use a simple journal or app—nothing too complicated—to write down how you feel before and after working out each day. This will help you spot any changes and get a better handle on what feels right for you.

And here's the beautiful part: don't be afraid to tweak your plan. If certain exercises aren't doing much for you or if you're feeling stuck, mix them up. Or if some workouts feel like they're becoming too easy, it may be time to ramp things up a little bit. Remember, the goal isn't to have a rigid routine that never changes—it's to find something that keeps you moving, happy, and mentally strong.

As you roll through these steps, you'll likely find that the more your workout plan progresses, the better you feel. And that's the whole point—to feel good, stay motivated, and keep that dopamine release flowing, so it supports not just your workouts but your everyday life.

In Conclusion

This chapter has shown us the powerful **relationship** between physical activity and dopamine, demonstrating how **exercise** can naturally support healthier and happier brains. By integrating **movement** into your daily life, you can reap both immediate and long-term **benefits** for your mood, focus, and overall well-being. Simple changes can make a big difference, especially when every step you take contributes to a happier you.

You've learned how exercise helps release dopamine in your brain, making you feel good and more **motivated**. You've discovered the short and long-term effects of physical activity on both mood and brain function. Various types of **exercise** like running and lifting weights each boost dopamine differently. You've seen examples of how mixing up your workouts can have an even greater effect on how good you feel. You've also picked up tips on incorporating small movements throughout the day and how these actions can keep you happier, longer.

Let these takeaways remind you that by simply getting up and moving, you can positively impact your **mind**. Take small steps to add more activity into your days. Equipped with these new **routines**, you can influence how you feel, bringing more smiles, energy, and balance into your daily life.

Chapter 8: Sleep and Dopamine Regulation

Have you ever wondered why a bad night's sleep seems to mess with your entire day—or even several days after? I know how it feels when one restless night throws everything off, and it turns out the **culprit** might be something you haven't thought much about: **dopamine**. There's a fascinating dance going on between how well you **sleep** and how your brain handles dopamine, which affects everything from your **mood** to your motivation.

You'll discover in this chapter just how **vital** sleep is for keeping your dopamine levels in check, like tuning an instrument so it can play harmoniously. And for those moments you can't help but catch a **power nap**... there's more to it than just "resting your eyes." By the end, you might start seeing sleep as your secret **weapon** for feeling balanced and sharp. Ready to get **started**?

Throughout this chapter, you'll learn about the intricate relationship between your sleep patterns and dopamine regulation. It's not just about feeling groggy after a bad night; it's about how your brain's chemistry is affected. You'll see why catching those Z's is crucial for maintaining a healthy dopamine balance, which in turn influences your daily life more than you might realize.

We'll dive into the science behind sleep's impact on your brain's reward system, and how it can make or break your day. You'll gain insights into why that afternoon siesta might be doing more good than you thought, and how to harness the power of sleep to keep your dopamine levels singing in tune.

So, buckle up and get ready to explore the fascinating world of sleep and dopamine. By the time you're done, you'll have a whole new appreciation for hitting the hay and might even find yourself looking forward to bedtime a bit more. Let's jump in and unravel the mysteries of sleep and its impact on your brain's feel-good chemical!

The Connection Between Sleep and Dopamine

Ever wake up from a terrible night's **sleep** and just feel... off? Maybe even a bit cranky, less motivated, or just plain sluggish? Well, there's a good chance your dopamine levels are playing a role here, and a lot of it comes down to how your sleep cycles are doing their thing. See, the way you go through different sleep stages can majorly impact dopamine production and how sensitive your receptors are to this all-important chemical. Imagine your brain as a busy kitchen, and dopamine is that secret sauce that makes everything run smoothly.

Let's talk about your sleep stages—these cycles from light sleep to deep sleep, and then the all-important REM. Each plays its own part in a kind of nightly dance that keeps dopamine levels in check. **Deep sleep**, for instance, is when your body goes into repair mode, cleaning up your brain and keeping dopamine levels balanced. Not enough of this, and you could be left with either too-few dopamine receptors or ones that aren't quite responsive enough. It's like when you miss a step while cooking—you notice things just don't come out right.

Speaking of these receptors—getting just the right amount of sleep sets them up to work effectively, ready to handle whatever life throws your way the next day. But when your sleep is disrupted? It messes with things. Kind of like skipping a meal—your body's just not going to give the best performance.

But let's ease into this next bit. The problem really shows up on those nights when you get far too little sleep. It's no surprise that missing out on enough shut-eye affects dopamine in all sorts of bad ways. Without sufficient sleep, these carefully regulated dopamine systems go haywire. Your **reward** processing? Totally thrown out of whack. And what does that mean for you? Well, simply put, you're more likely to find yourself reaching out for that extra cup of coffee or craving sugary snacks. You're not responding to rewards and motivation properly because sleep decided to take a back seat— throwing your dopamine system completely out of balance.

It's not just the quantity of sleep but also the type of sleep you're getting that matters. You have those perfect few hours where **REM sleep** cycles are synced up nicely with deep sleep. Your brain gets the right kind of bath it needs to function optimally, processing these dopamine pathways, making sure sensitivity is dialed in just where it needs to be. But if your sleep is fragmented, interrupted multiple times during the night, your dopamine system anticipates survival priority—chasing quick bursts of energy over long-term gains. That's how lack of sleep disrupts your drive, reward-seeking behavior, and even mood.

Now, wouldn't it be handy to see how this all plays out in an easy, visual manner? Introducing the "Sleep–Dopamine Harmony Chart"—a simple yet powerful tool to illustrate how different sleep stages come into play with dopamine activity. The idea is to match each type of sleep—with REM weighing in hardest—to dopamine production, distribution, and receptor sensitivity.

When you have an uninterrupted five 90-minute sleep cycles throughout the night, ranging from light sleep (where dopamine regulation stays generally minimal but consistent) to deep sleep (the repair and maintenance of dopamine firing and receptor efficiency), things connect the way they should. But skim on a few cycles, or most importantly that REM stage, and the whole harmony shatters. It's pretty much like trying to finish a **puzzle** with every fifth piece missing—you might get something resembling the whole picture, but you'll always know something critical is out of place.

This chart gives you a step-by-step visual insight into why decent sleep gives dopamine the green light to work at its best while the lack of deep or continuous sleep turns things chaotic. When what goes on down at the **molecular** level starts affecting how you feel and act each day, you come to realize sleep isn't just fluff. It's the cozy quilt that carefully stitches your dopamine together. So, the next time you find yourself thinking, "Oh, five hours will be enough," think again. Your dopamine—and your future self—will thank you.

Circadian Rhythms and Dopamine Production

Your body knows more about time than you might think. It doesn't just wake you up or make you sleepy; it actually has its own built-in **clock**, known as the circadian rhythm. But here's the cool part—not only does this clock help with sleep, but it also affects how your brain releases **dopamine** throughout the day.

This internal clock is like that background track in a movie. You might not always notice it's there, but it subtly guides everything that comes next. Think of the dawn or dusk, when sunlight triggers certain biological processes. Dopamine isn't just hanging around waiting to be used whenever you're low on energy or feeling bored. Oh no—it follows its own schedule, synced up with your body's sense of time. For example, dopamine levels **spike** in the morning as soon as you open your eyes. No wonder everyone feels that rush of motivation when the day is just beginning. This chemical spike gives you that oomph to tackle whatever's on your plate.

As the day rolls on, the timing of dopamine release influences everything from concentration to **emotion**. By early afternoon, when that heavy slump kicks in, yup, there's less dopamine pooling in your brain. That's why naps or a refreshing walk often do wonders—they're working to balance your energy with your natural dopamine dips. But here's where it gets interesting. Towards the evening, dopamine decreases, which encourages your body to start winding down.

When your schedule aligns with your body's circadian clock, your mood and **motivation** levels naturally ebb and flow like the tides— they follow a steady, predictable, and healthy pattern. But what if you don't stick to this rhythm?

Let's talk about the chaos that happens when that rhythm is thrown off. Whether you're pulling an all-nighter or clocking in odd hours, messing up your circadian rhythm can knock your dopamine levels right off track. When your sleep patterns are irregular, your mood usually takes a hit, right? Nothing seems quite right the next day— motivation feels miles out of reach, and getting through simple tasks feels like dragging a heavy weight. You're less motivated, flat-out tired, moody... maybe irritable too. It's not your fault—it's just daylight saving time and whatever other life events that shake up your sleep that take dopamine beautifully out of tune.

Over time, if this disruption keeps going, dopamine production can get all mixed up, which might even lead to more serious mood-related issues. Consider your body's timing like a band playing together. When everyone plays their part on time, the whole thing sounds harmonious. Mess up the timing even a little, though... chaos.

Still, all is not lost. You can keep this delicate dopamine dance on track by syncing up with your natural **clock**. How, you ask? Ever heard of a "Circadian-Aligned Dopamine Schedule"? It's not nearly as complicated as it sounds, but more like treating your brain like a garden. Every hour you're awake is like watering the soil. Following this schedule is about structuring your day in a way that nurtures the best possible dopamine production.

Start your day early if you can—when dopamine's naturally at its highest. Dive into the tasks that require the most effort first to ride that wave. As the day progresses, incorporate strategic breaks. In a meeting? Opt for standing or moving around a bit if it fits the environment. And when it comes to any screen time? It's especially helpful to limit the distractions towards the end of your day. Those evening hours are primed for winding down, not revving up.

By adapting your day-to-day routines in agreement with your circadian rhythm, you can ride along with the highs and lows of dopamine, instead of getting swept away. It's like planting seeds during the right season—you reap what's sown by working in harmony with your body's natural **rhythm**. Let your daily schedule embrace lifetime **alignment**, setting the stage for a balanced, fulfilling groove.

Sleep Hygiene for Optimal Dopamine Balance

Most of us know that a good night's sleep is crucial. But have you ever thought about how it ties into your **dopamine** levels? Picture this: you sleep poorly, you wake up feeling grumpy, and your motivation? Zilch. That's where sleep **hygiene** comes into play. It's all about creating the right habits to keep your dopamine, and by extension, your mood and motivation, in check. Let's dive into some tips that'll help you sleep better and, more importantly, take care of your dopamine levels.

Start simple. Set a regular **bedtime** and waking time—even on the weekends. Yeah, it sounds boring, but your body loves routine. It gets used to signals and works like a clock when you stick to a predictable schedule. This rhythm lets dopamine levels rise naturally in the morning, boosting your mood, and decline smoothly in the evening, preparing you for sleep. If you're all over the place with your sleep schedule, your dopamine won't know whether to keep you hyped up or mellow out. The result? You might struggle to fall asleep or, worse, wake up feeling like you never really slept.

And it's not just the timing—your **environment** is just as important. Keep your room dark. Sounds like nothing new, right? But seriously, block out all that artificial light creeping in. Your body processes light as a cue to stay awake because it thinks it's still daytime. Blue light in particular (you know, from your phone, tablet...anything with a screen) can mess up melatonin production, the sleep hormone that syncs well with dopamine to get you the rest you need. Put that phone away—or at least turn on the night mode if you really must have that last scroll.

Clean your room, too. It might seem weird to connect a tidy space with sleep quality, but an organized bedroom signals your brain that it's time to unwind. Avoid any work-related stuff in the same space—keep it chill, restful. Any clutter? It only raises your stress, not your dopamine.

Alright, now imagine you're settled into your consistent sleep schedule with a dark, cool, and meanwhile screen-less room. Let's connect this with the habits that can truly accentuate this effect... things like relaxation routines and avoiding certain pitfalls. Enter: Dopamine-Friendly Bedtime **Ritual**. Think of it as the ultimate wind-down plan.

Here's what you do. About an hour before bed, dim the lights around your home. Create a softer atmosphere. This helps with decreasing cortisol, the stress hormone that can blot out dopamine faster than you'd like. You might want to cap the day by having a warm bath; it's an oldie but goodie. It isn't just about relaxation; it helps drop your body temperature once you step out of the bath, subtly nudging your body and dopamine levels in the sleepy direction.

Next, consider **journaling**. Writing down your thoughts eases the mental clutter. That thing where your mind races with ideas, lists, worries—it's all fodder for keeping you awake. Getting it out on paper gives your brain the permission it's been waiting for to finally shut down. And a bonus? Reflect on the good stuff from the day— it builds up dopamine just before bed, setting you up for a night of positive charge restoration. Over time, this little nugget of positivity could mean you wake up with a more motivated, balanced state of mind.

Now, as you set yourself up for restful sleep with these habits, there's one last key: avoid the no-no's of sleep interference—like late-night caffeine or working out too close to bedtime. We love our coffee, but trade that PM mug for herbal tea. And if you're the midnight runner, switch it out with some morning outdoor time— which, by the way, also leads to a natural dopamine rise as sunlight hits your skin first thing.

It's all connected. Adopt, adjust, and stick with it. No rush. With better sleep, waking up will start to feel like a natural **high** each morning.

Napping and Its Effects on Dopamine Levels

Let's talk about naps. Some guys swear by them, like they're a magic reset button, while others fear they'll end up more tired than before. But what's the deal with how naps mess with your **dopamine**?

Here's the good news: naps can do wonders for your dopamine levels. A short snooze, say around 20 minutes, isn't just a quick rest. It's like a little **boost** for your brain's dopamine system. You won't just wake up feeling more alert; you'll likely feel more motivated. Dopamine's the stuff that helps you get things done, after all. That's why a properly timed nap can make you more ready to tackle whatever's next on your to-do list.

But there's a flip side. If you overdo it—let's say you nap way longer or nap too often—you can actually mess up your natural dopamine rhythms. You might wake up groggy or, worse, end up messing with your **sleep** cycles, which, let's be honest, just makes everything worse, especially come nighttime when you're supposed to be catching regular Zs.

Now, linking this up with how you can schedule your naps for the best results: **timing** is everything. You're not looking for long, luxurious sleeps in the middle of the day but rather, short, deliberate naps that serve a purpose—rebounding that dopamine to give you a quick reboot.

Mid-afternoon, like between 1 and 3 PM, tends to be prime nap territory. That's when your body's natural rhythm, called the **circadian** rhythm, dips. Subconscious yawns? That's your body waving a white flag. A nap during this time can give you a quick dopamine boost just when you start to feel that midday slump.

Something to remember: Nap strategically. You don't want to wreck your night's sleep, so avoid late afternoon or evening naps. Those are just going to make it harder for you to fall asleep later, throwing off all those natural rhythms your brain depends on.

Which leads us nicely into the kind of magic formula for napping—what we'll call the "**Strategic** Napping Protocol."

You might want to keep your naps to around 10-20 minutes. This keeps you in light sleep, so you don't fall into deep stages that might leave you feeling sluggish. If you've got an insane workload or feel all those incoming tasks piling up, try a "full cycle nap," roughly 90 minutes. This allows your brain to complete a sleep cycle, but that's pushing it in terms of time—more like an emergency restart option.

To really power this up as your dopamine-calming tactic, think about your surroundings. Grab a dark room, avoid any bright lights sneaking in. White noise or quiet background on your phone helps too. The idea is to give yourself no **distractions** so your mind can actually rest up and give you that quick, dopamine rebuild you're after.

So whether you're just looking to get back on balance during your nine-to-five or running on low fumes because of that sleep-thinning habit you cultivated, give napping a stronger look. Better sleep means better **dopamine** control, and that could change how you power through your day.

Practical Exercise: Developing a Sleep-Optimizing Routine

Taking a good, hard look at how you **sleep** these days—yeah, it's not the most fun thing to do. But it's where you start. Ask yourself: When do you actually hit the sack, and how long do you lounge around in bed looking at your phone before nodding off? Do you wake up a bunch of times during the night? You need to get real about what's messing with your sleep, whether it's late-night candy bingeing, noises, or even those cute, but unhealthy, all-nighters you pull every so often. This isn't about making you regret your habits—everyone's got sleep stuff to fix—it's about understanding what pieces you've got in your sleep puzzle so you can organize them better.

Now that you see the spots where your sleep routine could use some work, it's time to deal with step two: setting up a sleep **schedule**. Your body has a clock—a natural one—that knows when it's ready to knock out and when to get up. When you constantly confuse it with late-night Netflix or random naps, your body starts to lose it. So yeah, plan an actual bedtime. One you stick to pretty much every night so your body can fall into a pattern. And wake up at the same time too, even on weekends. I know, sounds tough, but consistency is where the magic happens. The more you stick to the schedule, the better you'll notice your body (and your mood, thanks to **dopamine**) falling into line.

Since we're on the topic, think of creating a pre-sleep routine like making a kid calm down before bedtime—except the kid here is you. Start winding down earlier in the evening doing stuff that tells your brain it's time to slow things down. Listen to calming music or read something, as long as it's not on your bright phone screen. By dimming the lights, putting on comfy sleepwear, and maybe sipping some warm tea that doesn't have caffeine (chamomile, anyone?), you're setting the mood—literally—for rest. Your body begins to associate these chill cues with preparing to sleep, helping to ramp down levels of that high-strung dopamine that's got you amped up.

On top of that routine, the place you sleep in has a huge impact. Take a glance around where you lay your head every night—there might be some things you need to tweak. While that comfy **mattress** is great, making sure your room is at a good, cool temperature matters too. Any light sources should be as close to gone as possible—yes, that means blackout curtains and shutting off those pesky blinking electronics. Quietness is gold, so think about earplugs or a white noise machine if your space tends to get loud. Keep your room and bed just for sleep—your brain should walk into that space ready to relax, not feel distracted by, I dunno, work projects or a pile of clothes needing folding.

While we're at it, let's not ignore how important **light** is during the day. It's not just about bedtime—your brain takes cues from daylight too. Getting good sunlight in the mornings helps set your inner clock, motivating your body to fall into a fun loop of waking and sleeping on cue. Come night, you've got to do the opposite and avoid screens that shoot bright blue light, which confuses your brain and stops melatonin, your natural chill-out hormone, from making the rounds. You want melatonin—it greases the wheels for dopamine to kick back into balance.

And of course, there's the old but trusty **mindfulness** trick. Bring in a little meditation or deep breathing before bed to calm your mind. Just a few breath cycles can ease your racing thoughts and pave the way to better quality sleep—no expensive gadgets needed. Start small. Maybe five deep breaths in bed, folding them into your routine until your body starts relaxing as soon as head meets pillow. Some of this will feel weird at first, but once it clicks, you'll see sleep becoming more natural.

Honestly, that's a lot already. But we're not done till you pin down how all of this is working for you. **Tracking** your sleep quality and how you feel during the day will let you really see what's up with your dopamine levels. Do you notice it getting easier to stay focused? Less moody? Start keeping a simple sleep diary or use one of those basic sleep-tracking apps to check how your nights are going. If this plan doesn't seem to be quite clicking, or if you're waking groggy, it's a sign to change things up a bit—adjust your bedtime, tweak that pre-sleep wind-down routine, or even add a little more sunlight to your mornings. Keep tweaking those gears till they fit just right.

Stick to these steps, and over time, you'll craft a sleep routine that not only feels natural but also strengthens that tricky balance between getting restful sleep and keeping your **dopamine** on a steady roll. Sweet dreams, right?

In Conclusion

This chapter has shown a strong connection between **sleep** and **dopamine**, revealing how the quality of your shut-eye directly impacts your body's ability to maintain balanced dopamine levels. By understanding and applying the guidelines provided, you've got the tools to boost both your **sleep** and **mood**, helping you feel better and stay more **motivated** each day.

You've seen how sleep cycles can affect dopamine levels in your brain, and the ways sleep deprivation can mess with dopamine production, making you feel less rewarded by positive things. You've also learned about the importance of tuning into your body's internal clock and its impact on dopamine levels.

This chapter has given you some solid tips for improving **sleep hygiene** to naturally maintain a healthier dopamine balance. You've also discovered that napping can be helpful, but it requires careful timing to support mood and brain health.

Now it's time to take what you've learned here and put it into practice daily. Your body's natural rhythms and proper sleep habits are like a dream team, working together to help you feel happier and more **energetic**. By making better sleep a priority, you're ensuring that your dopamine levels stay balanced, leading to more positive experiences and greater **motivation** as you tackle each new day!

So, go ahead and give your sleep the attention it deserves. Your brain will thank you, and you'll be setting yourself up for a more rewarding and upbeat life. Sweet dreams and happy dopamine balancing!

Chapter 9: Self-Regulation Strategies

Have you ever found yourself chasing that next rush—constantly caught in a cycle of feeling high, then low, over and over? I know what it's like, and trust me, it's totally **exhausting** after a while. But did you know there's a way to take **control** before it takes hold of you? In this chapter, I'll guide you through a path that puts the power back in your hands. You'll find yourself understanding more about how to **manage** your ups and downs, literally through physical **boundaries** and time-based actions.

I'm not just throwing around ideas here. No, every tip you'll come across can be easily **applied** to your daily routine. By the end of this, you'll be ready to craft your very own personal **plan**—and maybe even enjoy your high points a bit more without getting swallowed up by another crash. You, yes you, can **own** this!

You'll discover practical strategies to help you **regulate** your emotions and behaviors. These aren't just theoretical concepts; they're real-world techniques you can start using right away. From setting up physical reminders to creating time-based routines, you'll learn how to take charge of your emotional rollercoaster.

Remember, it's not about eliminating all the highs and lows—it's about finding a balance that works for you. You'll learn how to ride the waves without getting swept away, and how to make the most of your energy without burning out.

So, are you ready to take the reins? Let's dive in and explore how you can become the master of your own emotional landscape. Trust me, the view from the driver's seat is much better than being along for the ride.

Physical Boundaries for Dopamine Control

Setting up physical **boundaries** is crucial for managing your dopamine. It's like realizing your kitchen blender has five settings, but you've always used just the one that makes your smoothie too watery or too thick. The right setting—creating a space that respects your brain's craving for dopamine—makes all the difference. You live in a world where **distractions** are everywhere. Your phone, that bag of chips, or even the endless to-do lists. Each one triggering the blissful release of dopamine, that little chemical messenger of pleasure. Sounds great, right? But when you give in too often— bam!—you lose control. You end up seeking those "pleasures" not because they're good for you, but just because they're within reach. So, boundaries. Yeah, they exist for a reason, and they're not just for keeping noisy neighbors out of your yard. They help you stay focused, sane even, by reducing those random dopamine triggers.

Physically control what's within your sight, touch, or smell. Want to read more and binge less? Don't just think it; do it. Push the TV remotes and screens out of reach. Stash your phone in another room when it's bedtime. You don't need a lock-and-key situation to build these boundaries, although go for it if it helps. One guy gave his bed a rule: just sleep, nothing else. His friends thought he was nuts—a 'bed mission' they called it—but it sure worked. Sleep time went up, mindless browsing went down. The bed was now a dopamine trigger for sleep, like Pavlov's bell is to dogs. It might sound boring, but it's reliable. Plus, boring equals less clutter in dopamine paradise.

Now, onto the fun part: designing your **environment** for dopamine sanity. There's a trick or two here that, oddly enough, fit the energy bill too since you really should move that desk closer to that window anyway. Where you put things seriously affects how often you'll reach for them. Flip the placement of items like a mischievous elf turned minimalist designer—leave your book on the coffee table and nudge your phone back one room. It's like putting the ice cream in the storage space above the fridge—nobody likes bending for that long. Distracting stuff should be harder to get, more mindful reward stuff easier to reach. Micro-movements creating micro-habits, but they kinda feel like small wins.

Time to talk logistics. Enter "Dopamine-Conscious Space **Organization**" on stage. Think of this method as tidying up with purpose rather than vanity. You'll go after low-hanging fruit first— the bad behavior-hall-engines, we'll call them. That office stance creating the tortured tilt toward checking every beep alert right in front of you? That stops today. Where you plop yourself down matters. Arrange your desk so your **focus** stays on real work, not doom-scrolling every break. Give your eyes easy access to relaxing scenery, not productivity sidetracks. Staring at papers is one thing, but noticing fuzz on a picture in the corner until it's familiar just won't do.

Apply the principle everywhere else: Fridge? Stock it top-down with healthyish stuff at eye level—fruit front and center is better than cookies. Bedside table? Half the stuff there probably doesn't help your evening slump into comforting sleep—replace the techno-gadget dust collectors with an actual book or maybe a dim-lit alarm clock telling Hollywood sunrise time. Not rocket science at any stretch, feels obvious even. Yet, you've now purposely shaped little shrines to your intention.

With the environment you've just reshuffled, **distractions**, blessings, and **habits** ease or challenge differently. Don't be surprised if this makes something click inside you. Physical boundaries give you more emotional space, which—though barely harnessed it—also improves that ability to resist lying to yourself about wasting your evening after a peep at yet another meme fix. Sorta makes you wonder what form naturally follows the dopamine-behavior elephant you've just led through this small funnel...

And within that perfectly realigned space, everything stays just that—balanced, as curated as Marie Kondo's streamlined "joyful possessions," controlling **dopamine** release gets sorted too. How fitting.

Time-Based Strategies for Regulation

Ever find yourself **juggling** countless tasks only to feel drained by the end of the day? You're not alone. It's easy to get swept up in the rush, and there's something about those little dopamine hits that make you chase one high after another. But how can you keep this in check without burning out? Enter time-based methods for managing your dopamine stimulation. Let's kick things off with some strategies that'll help you create a **balanced** routine while still having time for those rewarding activities that make you feel great.

Managing your daily **schedule** doesn't have to be a chore, and you don't have to cut out those things that light you up completely. The trick is learning how to spread out dopamine-stimulating activities so they don't overwhelm you. Think of it this way: if you keep reaching for sweet snacks all day long, eventually, you'll feel that sugar crash. Your body has gone through the thrill so much that even your absolute favorite treat doesn't hit the same way. In the same sense, if you keep bouncing around from one exciting task to the next without reprieve, your mind doesn't get the chance to reset. The secret sauce here is **timeboxing** each activity—basically, setting aside dedicated chunks of time for specific tasks, both mundane and thrilling. By doing so, you allow your brain the downtime to recharge. Even 10 to 15 minutes of quiet between tasks can do wonders. You're still letting yourself enjoy the buzz when it comes along, but without that exhausting burnout.

But sometimes, you might find that the usual tricks aren't enough. It's one standby after another without anything changing — that's where scheduled dopamine "fasts" work their magic. Okay, "fast" might sound dramatic, but it's less extreme than you think. You're not cutting out all fun for good. Instead, you're stepping back—just temporarily. When you've pushed your dopamine triggers too much, stepping away can reset your **sensitivity**. Maybe that's shelving social media for a weekend or cutting out that binge-watching habit for a day. It's like hitting the reboot button for your brain. The goal is pretty simple: silence or low-stimulation activities that allow your dopamine receptors a chance to rest. Fatigue fades away, and you're left with renewed enthusiasm for the things that you're kind of numb to right now. Plus, believe it or not, by giving yourself that lull, you're stockpiling all the good feelings for when you finally hop back in. So, if Monday blues have shifted into Tuesday gloom, consider pressing pause for a day or two... give yourself the timeout your system craves.

Sure, talking about schedules and dopamine fasts is valuable, but there's a torchbearer product that ties it all together—call it the "Dopamine Time-Boxing Method." Think of this method as having your cake, eating it, but not stuffing down the whole thing in one go. By setting specific periods for shorter & long-term activities within your day (from work to that leisure scroll of your phone), you allow a **rhythm** that keeps things exciting without overflowing. You could time blocks for focused creative work sheeted with bits of buffer slotted in for things like mindfulness tasks. This one-two dance keeps your actions in motion, leaving enough slack for rejuvenation. The result? You achieve your goals while balancing the highs.

Juggling priorities and protecting mental zing might sound tricky. Yet it boomerangs back to one essential act: pacing yourself. By weaving management strategies like this into your daily hustle, stumbling onto boredom or burnout becomes a distant memory. The best thing? Once you start penning down these habits into your days, you'll notice a more **balanced** feeling that was probably missing before.

Categorical Approaches to Dopamine Management

Alright, let's chat about **dopamine**. You know it's like the fuel for your brain's drive, right? So, how about sorting out your daily activities based on their dopamine "cost" to help keep everything in balance? It's kinda like organizing your pantry—you've got the sweets, salty snacks, the healthy stuff, and maybe a few treats for special moments. Doing this with dopamine-related activities helps manage your excitement and keeps you on track when life's pulling you in every direction.

Picture grouping activities into categories based on how they affect your **motivation**, happiness, and calmness. Toss low-dopamine activities like reading a novel or chatting with a buddy into one pile, save medium-impact things like playing a game or attending a chill meeting for another. And finally, stack those high-dopamine kicks where they belong—stuff like scrolling social media, gossiping, or binge-watching that TV show could all go in the "handle with care" category. Mixing these up intentionally helps you decide what's worth a big splash of dopamine and when to settle for something that won't drain or overstimulate you completely. It's like planning a diet so you feel satisfied without all that unhealthy binging.

Now, let's talk about a **dopamine budget**. Always chasing that next high! Sounds fun, sure, but it can be a slippery slope. That's where this budgeting idea comes into play. By setting aside specific times in your day when you say, "I'll indulge this much excitement, and no more for now," you create a smart way to manage all the highs and lows. Think of it as giving yourself flexibility but within a safe framework. Just like you wouldn't blow your paycheck on fast food (well, maybe sometimes, but it's not great long-term), you wouldn't want to spend an entire afternoon glued to social media just for those little dopamine hits.

Create a **budget** that leaves room for everything—the necessary but not-so-thrilling activities alongside those electric, dopamine-spiking experiences. For example, decide on your screen time after handling other obligations or choose a day to skip the chaotic errands and instead invest in conversations with your buddies that keep you excited, but in a healthy way. This budgeting shows where your priorities lie and helps keep your dopamine levels in check—even when life throws that unpredictable stress your way. Imagine not only surviving but thriving in a distracting world—feeling clear-headed instead of scattered because you've got a plan to control each surge of excitement.

Now, here's my mild obsession—the "**Dopamine Category System**." Sorting activities? Check. Managing budgets? Double check. But how do you categorize your approach to every source of excitement or happiness in life? Let's break it down. You've got a system that governs your extremes: "Lent-to" involves detoxing, abstaining from that high-stakes reward, whether that's from the endless delight of online videos or binge-watching your favorite series. Lesson two—high reward means caution, looking at it scientifically. Yeah, that Netflix series might sound thrilling, but do you *need* that much dopamine in one go? Could you stream gradually, a slow-and-steady race toward satisfaction?

Then there's the mid-level stuff—where it's easy to restore yourself without going overboard. Think biking (maybe in a spot with no phone reception), pilates, or scheduled fun like family game nights. These keep you flexible, aware of pleasure sources, but anchor you without oversaturating your excitement receptors. The system fits right into life and paints a picture: activities tied to joy, plans tied to budget, aiming for zero burnout in a healthy framework of choices. It simplifies your options, pushing you toward balanced energy inputs and protecting you from impulse aftermath or unsustainable excitement spirals.

It's a fresh start—managing dopamine this way changes how you think about temptation, resetting your approach to stretch minimal enjoyment more meaningfully or gain overall function through clearer perception. Integrate **lifestyle changes**, add those touching moments within conscious opt-in periods, embracing both sides yet favoring grounded practice as a dopamine budgeting strategy to prevent wild spin-outs or silently overindulging cravings.

So as you go through your day, ready to tackle a task or give yourself a moment to chill (or rev up!), remember this dopamine budgeting trick and categorization helps you stay grounded, accountable, and ultimately satisfied without maxing out your dopamine reserves or falling into depletion cycles. See it as less about redlining and more about learning self-stimulation that's proportional to bright enlightenment rather than getting stuck in a burn-out cycle. It's about managing those dopamine-laden activities that lure you in, and finally reaching a balance that favors realistic devotions and measured productivity through consistent, well-paced growth.

Happy dopamine mission, bro! Keep it balanced, keep it real, and enjoy the ride.

Implementing Self-Regulation in Daily Life

Self-regulation—sounds like something fancy and complicated, right? But really, it's just learning to **control** those impulses, especially the ones that give you that instant hit of dopamine. You know, the ones that pull you towards checking your phone every few minutes or grabbing that extra piece of chocolate. It all starts with **self-awareness**, recognizing how and when you tend to go hunting for dopamine. And believe me, we all do.

Right now, think about your typical day. How much of it is spent hunting for that quick buzz? Whether it's popping on social media, mindlessly scrolling through reels, or just zoning out with some meaningless content. That's your dopamine talking. The more you catch yourself in these moments, the easier it gets to manage them. Make it a habit to pause and ask yourself, "Why am I doing this?" That simple question can pull the brakes on automatic behaviors. You start noticing a pattern—or a whole bunch of them. Maybe it's stress, boredom, or just habit that leads you down this path. Name that pattern, stare it in the face, and call it what it is.

Once you're aware, it's time to put up some **roadblocks**. I know, easier said than done, right? But that's where personal cues and reminders come into play. How many times have you thought to yourself, "I'm just gonna check this one thing," and suddenly, an hour has flown by? Yep, I've been there too. But let's toss some sand in the gears of that habit. Start small: put sticky notes near your temptations (laptop, fridge, you name it). Little messages like, "Do you really need this right now?" or "45 minutes to boredom isn't gonna kill you." These can be weird at first, maybe even annoying. But eventually, they become your mental speed bumps.

What about **triggers**? Part of this process is recognizing where all those dopamine-seeking moments stem from and throwing in some strategic interruption points. Is it when you walk through the door after work? How about while sitting on the couch after dinner? If so, find a healthier activity to jump into instead—something engaging enough that satisfies the urge but doesn't send you spiraling into more dopamine hits. Replace scrolling with, say, a quick walk outside or even a chat with a friend or family member. The idea is, when you get that itch, you don't scratch it the same old way.

But even with all these precautions, self-regulation is never a set-it-and-forget-it scenario. You've gotta keep tabs on your **progress**. That's where the "Dopamine Self-Check Technique" swoops in. It's not rocket science; it's more like your little mental bat signal. Every so often—could be every week or even daily—sit down and honestly evaluate how you've been managing things. Here's a quick rundown:

• Ask yourself—is your **mood** better? Worse? The same? What behaviors have shifted, and which, well, still need work?

• Rethink your cues—Do your sticky notes work? Are they just getting ignored? If they need a refresh, go ahead—modify them or move them somewhere more in-your-face.

• Adjust as necessary—It's not about getting it perfect. It's about getting it a little bit better each day.

None of this happens overnight, of course. Take it slow, give yourself some grace, and lean into this **technique**. It's a simple check-in but powerful enough to keep your dopamine-seeking habits in check, little by little. After a while, you'll find that self-regulation doesn't have to be restrictive or hard—just a sidekick helping you stay **balanced** in all that day-to-day chaos.

Practical Exercise: Crafting Your Self-Regulation Plan

There's no one-size-fits-all strategy when it comes to keeping **dopamine** in check. But you can start by paying attention to what revs your brain's dopamine engine. Think of those **triggers**—whether it's scrolling on your phone way past bedtime or reaching for another cup of coffee when you're already jittery. Identifying these moments is the foundation of your self-regulation plan.

Spend just a bit of time each day noticing patterns in when you're most likely to chase that next dopamine hit. This might happen when you're stressed, trying to avoid something unpleasant, or just plain bored. Jot down what comes to mind, especially when you catch yourself lost in activities that leave you feeling more foggy than fulfilled. Seeing it on paper makes it real—it's not just in your head anymore. It's a real thing you can work with. And from there, once you understand the forces at play, you'll find you're not as helpless as you might've thought.

Once you know the landscapes of your dopamine spikes, you need some go-to **alternatives** for moments of temptation. The idea is simple: when you're stuck in that limbo where you're fighting the urge to, say, waste half an hour in front of a screen, you'll already have a list of other stuff you can do instead. The key here is to choose things that give you a different kind of satisfaction—they might not light up your brain quite as much in the short term, but they're easier on the self-control reserves.

You could try doing something with your hands like cooking or gardening, or maybe taking a walk or diving into a good book. It's about finding joy in the slower, quieter moments rather than constantly chasing highs. Put pen to paper—or fingers to keyboard—and actually list these activities. Stick the list somewhere visible; think of it as a **toolbox** ready for whenever your dopamine levels get a bit too rowdy.

Alright, you've got awareness and alternatives. But without **boundaries**, all that knowledge can just vaporize in a moment of weakness. So you're going to want to set firm, clear limits on how you're engaging with the things that amp up your dopamine. This isn't about abstinence—relax, I'm not telling you to go cold turkey on all your favorite things—but a bit of moderation, for sure.

Maybe it's deciding you're only going to check social media for fifteen minutes after lunch. Anything outside that window? Sorry, it's a no-go. Or you could reserve your most dopamine-driving snacks for weekends only. A good rule of thumb: if something's got you hooked, set more limits—like a leash on a dog eager to chase every squirrel in sight. Without those boundaries, it's far too easy to get tricked by your urges.

Once you have your limits, you're not done just yet. Doing this without rebooting your entire **routine**? Yeah, that'd be tough. Integrating these strategies into a daily flow is the real key to making it actually work. Begin with the stuff you really have to do—work, caregiving, chores, whatever's on your day-to-day script. But build into that script new slots that invite lower-dopamine activities sandwiched in with your essentials.

Maybe the mornings start with news (but only 10 minutes max—remember those limits!). Later, once work piles up and you're tempted to beat the slump with late afternoon phone-checks? Swap it for a quick breather outside or five minutes stretching. Creating such a mix allows you to tick off your must-dos and helps recalibrate your brain away from addiction to constant rewards.

Tracking works like a personal scoreboard, ensuring you're not just drifting aimlessly. Start simple—don't overcomplicate it. Maybe it's just noting down an X on a paper calendar each day when you stick to your plan, or using an app to track when you've hit your goals. Rewards don't hurt either. We're not talking anything huge here—maybe a small treat or some other indulgence—a way to reinforce those smart choices.

But let's be real... Life happens, and from time to time, you might slip back into old habits. That's not what spells ruin—what really matters is your ability to **bounce back**. Think up a personal strategy for relapses ahead of time. If you suddenly find yourself diving headfirst into a dopamine overload, don't judge yourself too harshly. Just reset. Dedicate a time or a day to review what went wrong. Where did your plan falter? Once you know, patch the holes and get right back on track. Even missteps are part of the process.

Last but far from least—you gotta check in on yourself. Regular **check-ins**—maybe every Sunday night?—help gauge how well your self-regulation plan is working. Ask yourself things like, "Am I slipping into any old patterns?" or "Is this plan still working for me?" Adjustments are fair game if needed. It's not set in stone—you get to keep tweaking your plan until it clicks.

In Conclusion

This chapter equips you with **actionable steps** for managing dopamine levels in your life by introducing essential strategies and techniques. It zeroes in on how creating physical boundaries, optimizing your **environment**, being mindful of time and tasks, and practicing self-awareness can influence how you manage dopamine triggers effectively. You've seen a wide range of approaches to regulate and **balance** your dopamine for better mental and emotional well-being.

You've learned about:

• The importance of using physical spaces to create boundaries and manage stimuli effectively

• How designing your surroundings can help regulate dopamine levels

• Techniques like "Time-Boxing" to aid in managing daily tasks and balancing activities that engage dopamine

• How organizing your day with deliberate "dopamine budgets" can help in self-regulation

• Strategies to become more aware of and adjust your environment and daily practices for healthier dopamine management

This chapter serves as your **guideline** to crafting and administering practical steps that will not only help regulate dopamine in your life but also enrich your daily experiences. Feel **empowered** to apply these lessons so that you can go forth and build a lifestyle that supports balance, productivity, and overall well-being. Keep **experimenting** and fine-tuning, because small changes in how you manage dopamine today can make a big difference tomorrow.

Remember, it's all about finding what works for you. Don't be afraid to tweak these strategies to fit your unique lifestyle and needs. The key is to stay **consistent** and patient as you implement these changes. Before you know it, you'll be on your way to a more balanced and fulfilling life, with your dopamine levels working for you rather than against you. So, go ahead and take that first step – your future self will thank you for it!

Chapter 10: Dopamine Fasting

Have you ever felt like everything around you is just too much? That there's always a new **distraction** pulling you in every direction? I get it. I've been there too. This chapter is all about taking a step back from the noise and helping you, one day at a time, find that quiet space in your mind where real **clarity** happens. Think of it as hitting the reset button—one that's within your grasp. By the end of this chapter, you'll not only understand *why* it's important but also *how* to do it. So, as we dive in, think about what a little **breathing room** might look like in your life. Curious yet? Let's see how this chapter can get you there.

You're probably familiar with the constant **buzz** of notifications, the endless scroll of social media, and the never-ending stream of **entertainment** at your fingertips. It's no wonder you might feel overwhelmed sometimes. But here's the thing: you have the power to take control. **Dopamine fasting** isn't about depriving yourself; it's about giving yourself the gift of **focus** and **peace**.

Imagine a day where you're not constantly reaching for your phone, where you're fully present in each moment. Sounds refreshing, right? That's what we're aiming for. By the time you finish this chapter, you'll have the tools to create that experience for yourself.

So, buckle up, my friend. We're about to embark on a journey that could change the way you interact with the world around you. Are you ready to discover how a little less can actually give you so much more? Let's dive in and explore the world of dopamine fasting together.

Understanding the Concept of Dopamine Fasting

So, what exactly is **dopamine** fasting? You might've heard people talking about taking a break from almost everything—TV shows, social media, even food. And really, it's about hitting the pause button on things that usually give you a quick rush of pleasure. The idea behind dopamine fasting is to **reset** your brain's reward system. Kinda similar to when you overwater a plant and have to hold off to let it recover. Your brain loads up on dopamine every time you check your phone or eat a sugary snack, and after a while, it's nearly drowning in it. So dopamine fasting comes in to dry things out, so your brain can go back to its natural state. A little breathing room, if you will.

During a dopamine fast, you intentionally avoid certain **activities** that give you that jolt of instant good feelings. The sorts of things that usually get in the way of long-term happiness. We're talking about the endless scroll through social media, the binge-watching, the snacking out of boredom—all those things. Instead of staying in that constant cycle of instant dopamine spikes, you take some time out. The hope is that after your break is over, you'll find joy in the simpler things again, like a paper-thin slice of apple, or a meaningful chunk of books. And yeah—it's not just a whims-of-the-moment fad. **Research** shows taking these fasts can bring your dopamine levels back to baseline, making it easier for you to appreciate everyday life more. And who doesn't want that?

But there's a catch. A lot of people misunderstand what dopamine fasting is, turning it into something it's not. It's not about cutting off everything pleasurable forever. Some people, though, get this wild idea that it's some **cleanse** where you have to shun everything fun. Endless spirals of drastic all-or-nothing thinking online do a lot of damage. Folks hear the term, freak out, and say they'll fast from anything enjoyable. But here's the deal—even dull activities can boost dopamine, not just the fun ones. That's why you can miss the

118

mark if you're not actually focusing on what drains your dopamine reserves the fastest.

Alright, let's clear up some of these confusions before they spook you away. You don't have to starve yourself of dopamine, abandon your pals, or live like a hermit. Here's the truth right in front of you.

• You don't have to give up everything that makes you smile. It's about controlling only those actions that overpower your brain with too much dopamine. Think **moderation**.

• It's not a long, harsh retreat with just you and your thoughts. Even with fasts, there are still limits. It's possible to include low-dopamine activities like reading or light walks.

• This doesn't mean you'll be alone. It just means taking control over habitual desires—choosing when to check out—while keeping yourself socially active.

• It's not just a polish on digital detox. Sure, turning off the screens helps. But this fasting probably requires you taking stock and stepping back from other habits too, like constant eating or everyday pleasantries you overdo.

This all aims to correctly reset your thoughts—getting some quick **peace** for your brain. Not to be ascetic, but to explore what's getting in the way of real **happiness** in life—and clean that clutter out. And by busting these myths, it clears the way to try dopamine fasting the right way... without the misunderstandings. Sounds more doable now, right?

Planning Your Dopamine Fast

So, you're thinking about doing a **dopamine fast**, huh? Good idea. It can actually help **reset** your brain's pleasure circuits, almost like giving them a well-deserved vacation. You might be wondering how long you should go for or just how intense this fast should be. That's where a little reflection comes in.

Start by asking yourself some questions. How much **stimulation** are you swamped with daily? If your life revolves around constant notification buzzes and keeping up with endless social content, a longer fast might be more effective. Though, don't overcommit. The last thing you want is to white-knuckle your way through something too extreme and then feel like throwing in the towel after a day. A weekend, maybe two days, is a good starter. But if you're feeling like dipping your toes in, an afternoon could also make a lot of difference. Just remember, this isn't about suffering or making yourself miserable, but about giving your mind some well-earned space to breathe.

Here's a trick: look at the areas you think need the most reset. If you're truly fed up with mindlessly scrolling all day, maybe cutting social media out should be the focal point. But if it feels like TV is your constant background noise, focus there. Tailor the fast to what **stimulates** you the most. Does it all feel too overwhelming? Consider starting with just a few hours and build up from there.

Now, let's talk about getting your head in the game. Because, honestly, prepping for this is half the battle. It requires a certain **mindset**. Going into this, understand that discomfort may come up because you're so used to distracting yourself. Reflect on why you're doing this. What do you hope to gain? Some peace? Greater clarity? More focus? Whatever that is, keep it in mind if you encounter any tough moments when the itch begins to start up. Having intention set before you go in helps a lot too.

Let's get practical for a second—clear your schedule. Going low-stimulation while needing to keep up with work emails or deadlines could blow up in your face. Pick a time when your responsibilities are low. You don't want constant pulls on your attention defeating the purpose of what you're trying to achieve. It's like trying to meditate in the middle of Times Square. Doesn't really work.

Finally, let's put everything down into your game plan. Think of this like your "Personalized Dopamine Fast **Blueprint**." Start by sketching out a layout of what you're going to avoid—no TV? Social media block? Reading only approved books? Keep it in writing, so your goal becomes something you can refer back to throughout. You can even throw in a list of approved activities—things you find calming, like walking, or journaling, or maybe just sitting in a cafe with a hot drink (without checking your phone). Just be sure to decide what content you're going to allow, that relates directly to your purpose, and stick with it. And somewhere in that blueprint, drop a **reward** in there—something nice but stimulating so you're not tempted afterward to binge on what you restricted.

By personalizing it, you make it yours. You avoid a one-size-fits-all mistake where you're attempting rules from someone else's fast that might not fit your life at all. You take a balanced approach that helps you gain the mental space you need without diving face-first back into habits you're really trying to pace back on. It's about rest, centering, and rediscovering a part of yourself. No major overhauls—just simple **clarity**.

Implementing the Fast Effectively

When you're doing a **dopamine fast**, it's not uncommon to run into annoying **cravings** or that all-too-familiar discomfort. You get that itch, almost like you miss the distractions you're trying to cut out. The thing is, those cravings are your brain's sneaky way of telling you that it really, really likes its usual dose of easy dopamine. Kind of like how you don't notice you're hungry until you hear your stomach growling... craving distractions is the brain's version of that. But, here's the kicker, cravings are temporary. And they get weaker the more you push through them.

One way to tackle these cravings is by having a **plan** ready before they even hit you. Maybe get rid of things that usually make you reach for your phone or your usual "fix" — like if you tend to check social media first thing in the morning, maybe don't keep your phone next to your bed. It's like trying to avoid cookies when you're on a diet. The less they're around, the easier it gets.

Another **strategy**? Find something to keep your hands busy. Throwing yourself into something with repetitive actions that don't need too much thinking can be grounding. Knitting, doodling, playing with a stress ball... whatever floats your boat. It kills that gap when the urge to click on something or scroll pops up. And, as an added bonus, it might even get you mindful for a minute or two.

Changing **activities** also helps refocus your attention. Like, when the urge comes, get moving — literally. A quick walk, even if it's just pacing around your living room, can be surprisingly effective in shaking off a craving. And if all else fails, simple breathing exercises are always in your toolkit. Deep breaths, in and out... things are usually less intense by the time you've done a few rounds. They don't just soothe, they help bring you back to the moment.

So, once you've got a handle on staying cool when discomfort shows up, pivot to keeping things in balance while you're fasting. The idea here is to engage your brain in ways that don't hijack your dopamine levels in the process. Simple tasks, like cleaning or organizing, can be incredibly satisfying without overloading your system. Ever notice how there's a weird sense of calm that comes once you've tidied things up? No flashy rewards, just a quiet sense of order.

You might also find value in **creative** pursuits. Painting, journaling, or even cooking something from scratch can be gratifying in a low-key way. Unlike social media or online shopping sprees, these activities require you to be directly involved — hardly passive. You're nurturing something slowly... giving time for a gradual sense of accomplishment to settle, instead of that instant high and crash.

Now, ensuring **success** during a dopamine fast involves getting things together — what some folks might call their "Dopamine Fast Survival Kit." And it's not about grabbing a bunch of stuff. It's more about setting up your environment in a way that makes fasting easier, less tempting, and ideally, more enjoyable.

Here are the must-haves:

• Physical Space: Creating a distraction-free zone. Just like how you wouldn't leave junk food out when on a diet, try doing the same with that phone or computer. Clean, uncluttered spaces reduce mental noise.

• Focused Activities: Have a go-to list of things that can occupy you when boredom hits. Books that have been on your shelf for a while, puzzles, or simple crafts are good options.

• Mindfulness Tools: Consider adding a few coping tools that help you stay present. Again, breathing exercises, guided meditation apps (even if using a phone), or just sitting still are incredibly effective. In fact, finding peace in stillness might end up being one of the most profound experiences during your fast.

• A Journal: Documenting your thoughts, feelings, or even just jotting down snippets of what's happening helps you ride through waves of irritation or temptation. Plus, it serves as a way to reflect on how the process is affecting you.

After all that preparation and a bit of **mindfulness**, you'll likely find the dopamine fast easier than expected. Sure, there will be moments when it feels tougher than you thought. But with the right tools and some patience, you'll get through it. Most importantly, this exercise refines your relationship with dopamine — where you take back some control, instead of letting distractions lead the dance every time.

Reintroducing Stimuli Post-Fast

So you've made it through a **dopamine fast**—those minimal-stimuli, slightly introspective days are now behind you. Kudos for sticking with it! But before you dive back into all the activities that give you that rush, it's crucial to be cautious and intentional about it. Why? Because, believe it or not, plunging headfirst into those old habits could send you right back to square one. And we don't want that, do we?

As the fast ends, the **lure of dopamine** might feel stronger than ever. But instead of going wild, you need to tread carefully. Think of your brain like a sponge that just dried out. Now, if you chuck it straight into a bucket of water—that's too much, too soon—guess what? It just soaks and overflows as if it's never been dry before. This means you could easily find yourself binge-watching a series or endlessly scrolling through social media in no time. Not to mention—ending a fast like this could wipe out all those **gains** you've worked hard for. So in simple terms, a controlled reintroduction helps you enjoy those activities again without getting hooked all over.

Alright, so now that you've got a rough idea of why you should take it slow, let's chat about how to use this **detox period** to make some long-haul changes in your routines. And spoiler alert—it's easier to do right now than you might think.

You've probably noticed some daily behaviors or activities during the fast that no longer seem as appealing. Maybe that endless loop of checking texts every five minutes doesn't seem as rewarding now. So while you're still in that zone, fresh from the fast, it's the perfect time to drop or alter those habits for the better. For example, consider using what's been filling your time more productively. If boredom set in and you found yourself reading a book or taking more walks, hang on to that. Replace your automatic reaction of grabbing your phone with something a bit more fulfilling. Before you know it, these little swaps will become part of your routine.

But let's be real—memories fade, fast or not. Sometimes, reverting back to comfort is too tempting. The pull of auto-pilot is real. The solution? A simple plan, something you can fall back on whenever the itch for a **dopamine hit** gets too strong.

Let's call it the "Post-Fast Dopamine Recalibration Plan." The idea here is pretty straightforward, but can go a long way in protecting your progress and steering clear from slipping back. First, mentally list out the activities you're going to reintroduce. Pick one, and only one, to start with. Spend some time with it; get back into it gradually. Ask yourself—did you find it as joyful as before? Or did its charm wane during your fast? Once you're comfortable, move onto the next activity. By taking things step by step, you lessen the chance of overwhelming yourself or flooding your brain with too much dopamine all at once.

If you feel that tell-tale urge to get lost in all your previous **distractions**, pump the brakes. Step back and revisit how the fast made you feel—more focused, settled, maybe even more creative? Let that good stuff guide you. It's okay to go back, but this time, do it with more control, more intention, while paying attention to what sensations crop up with each old habit revisited. Our goal here is steady-paced, not sprinting—and that's what will make your post-fast **dopamine levels** work with you, not against you.

Slowing down allows new, healthier habits to blossom as your go-to sources of satisfaction. Translate some of that extra focus into lasting changes. That way, your brain won't just start craving everything you were trying to avoid but rather, will start enjoying the slower, more intentional ways you engage with the world.

Practical Exercise: Preparing for Your Dopamine Fast

Before you **dive** into a dopamine fast, it's crucial to take a good, honest look at what's driving those little dopamine hits throughout your day. Think about it—your daily routine is probably peppered with all sorts of activities that give you a quick shot of pleasure, right? Scrolling through your social media feed, catching up on your favorite shows, munching on snacks, or even the constant ding of notifications—these are all prime suspects. And sure, each one might seem harmless on its own. But when you put them all together, they contribute to a cycle of craving more and more.

Consider how these activities really **affect** your day-to-day life. Do they disrupt your focus? Make you more restless when you actually need to get something done? Or maybe, they just make it harder to enjoy the simpler stuff, like having a chat with a friend or reading a book? Getting a grip on how these dopamine triggers play into your life requires a bit of self-reflection. It's about noticing patterns and understanding where your attention gets pulled. Only when you know what's feeding your dopamine cravings can you start to make a real change.

Once you've **identified** the major players in your dopamine game, it's time to figure out what you want out of your dopamine fast. Setting clear goals will keep you grounded and give you direction. Do you want to cut out certain habits completely or just tone them down? Maybe you're looking to improve focus or just feel more contented with the simple parts of life. You could even plan for multiple checkpoints or milestones to see your progress along the way. This isn't about making rules you're going to resent; it's about setting benchmarks that you actually care about.

Having goals also gives you something to hold onto—a **purpose**, if you will—during moments when the fast gets tough. You'll be able to remind yourself why you're pushing through the discomfort. Craft these goals realistically, almost like mental notes you'll glance at, rather than some high-pressure expectations. By knowing exactly what you're aiming for, you'll find it much easier to navigate through the fast without getting lost along the way.

At this point, you should be thinking of the nitty-gritty stuff. How long should your dopamine fast be? And how restrictive? There's no one-size-fits-all answer here. You could go hardcore and pare it down entirely for a day—some people do, and it works for them. Or, maybe a weekend off the grid without screens might make more sense for you. Watch out, though—starting off too aggressive might just make you, well, miserable. Sometimes an afternoon free from your main dopamine triggers is a good starting point. Just remember, this isn't set in stone. You can always tweak the length or level of restriction as you learn more about what works for you.

Pick right, and rest assured—it'll pay off in how you feel afterward. That's the key, isn't it? Finding the sweet spot where you **challenge** yourself without completely wiping out your willpower. That balanced approach helps lay the groundwork for a successful fast.

Moving forward, you'll want to create an **environment** that actually supports your dopamine fasting efforts. Think about it: your regular setting might just keep spurring you to give in. When planning a fast, preparing your space is a game changer. If your usual go-to's aren't easily accessible, it'll be that much easier to stay committed. This could mean putting your phone on 'Do Not Disturb,' or keeping tempting snacks out of sight. Heck, if watching shows is your kryptonite, maybe stash away your remote, too. Little tweaks like these ease the process. Eliminate the things that usually lure you in, and you'll find much less resistance, less 'OMGs, I need to check my phone,' and more 'Okay, I can do this.'

The next thing to think about? What are you going to do with all that free time? Without those typical dopamine-boosting activities, you might straight-up feel bored, antsy, even restless. This is why you need some chill, feel-good activities to fall back on—things that are low-key and don't flood your brain with happy chemicals. Reading a book you've wanted to pick up but never got around to, taking a nature walk, or even sketching something could come in handy. These activities might be a far cry from your regular "rush."

Still, they can be almost soothing, giving you something to focus on as you let the dopamine-driven cravings wear off.

Have a plan for when patches of boredom strike. Consider it a downtime **strategy**, if you will—gentle activities that ease you through the discomfort. Think of them as small rewards for toughness that doesn't break your fast's purpose.

One last thought: when tackling something like a dopamine fast, one of your most powerful allies is having someone in your corner. **Accountability** matters. A friend or even a loved one knowing what you're up to can stop you from slipping without meaning to. Honestly, consider finding a buddy who's down to do the fast with you. That way, you share the wins, struggles and keep each other going when it's tempting to give in. They might just text you in the middle of the fast and say, 'How's it going?' It's a surprising help and sometimes, that check-in is all you need to stay on track.

In these last moments before the fast begins, think a smidge about the other side of it. No rush, but you need to have a plan for when to bring dopamine-boosting activities back into your life. Don't let them hit you like a sock to the jaw after the fast ends. Instead, trickle them back in—a bit at a time. Savor activities that you'd usually speed through, truly experiencing them. The fast's whole point is to make you mindful, isn't it? This reentry phase seals everything you've learned and rounds off—the lid to your completed process.

Through clarity and preparation, everything you plan will help you steady the course of your fast and beyond it.

In Conclusion

Dopamine fasting is more than just a trendy idea—it's a thoughtful way to **recalibrate** your brain's response to pleasure and stimulation. This chapter has laid out the concept, its **benefits**, and how to make it work for you. Whether you're looking to decrease **distractions** or simply reset your mood, the practice **empowers** you to regain control over how you interact with daily stimuli.

In this chapter, you've learned about what dopamine fasting really means, rather than the common myths surrounding it. You've seen why setting clear **goals** makes the fast more effective and easier to maintain. You now know that planning ahead is crucial for managing cravings and avoiding pitfalls. You've discovered how simple, alternative activities can help balance brain chemistry during the fast. Lastly, you understand the importance of slowly reintroducing pleasure-inducing stimuli after the fast to sustain long-term benefits.

By now, you're **equipped** with not only the why but also the how of dopamine fasting. Applying these steps may seem challenging, but the **mindset** shift it brings can lead to a healthier, more mindful lifestyle. The next time you feel overwhelmed by digital distractions or maybe just out of sync, consider giving dopamine fasting a try. Who knows? It might be the **reset** you didn't know you needed.

Chapter 11: Goal Setting and Dopamine Motivation

Have you ever noticed how setting a **goal** can suddenly make you feel more energized? It's like a switch flips, right? That's exactly what happens when you get a taste of **Dopamine**—the chemical that gets your brain talking. In this chapter, we'll dig deep into how you can use this knowledge to your advantage. By the time you're done reading, this thing called 'Dopamine' won't just be some scientific term, it'll be your secret **weapon** for staying motivated.

Sometimes **goals** seem overwhelming, but there's a way to trick your brain into feeling good along the way, even with the little victories. You'll even learn how to **recover** when things don't go your way, without losing that vital **motivation**. By the end of this chapter, you'll be equipped with practical **tricks** that encourage your brain to keep pushing you forward, one Dopamine hit at a time.

You'll discover how to harness the power of this **chemical** to your advantage, turning it into a driving force behind your ambitions. Whether you're tackling a big project or just trying to build better habits, understanding how Dopamine works can be a game-changer. You'll learn how to break down your goals into manageable chunks, creating a series of small wins that keep you pumped up and moving forward.

But it's not all smooth sailing, right? Sometimes things go sideways, and that's where the real magic happens. You'll find out how to bounce back from setbacks without letting your **motivation** take a nosedive. It's all about reframing those obstacles and keeping your eyes on the prize.

So, buckle up, buddy. You're about to embark on a journey that'll transform the way you think about goal-setting and motivation. By the time you finish this chapter, you'll have a toolbox full of strategies to keep your Dopamine flowing and your goals within reach. Let's dive in and unlock the secrets to staying motivated, one Dopamine boost at a time!

The Science of Goal-Oriented Dopamine Release

Let's talk about **dopamine**. You know that rush you get when you're excited about something coming up? Yeah, that's dopamine doing its thing. It's not just your average feel-good chemical—it's a real **motivator**. When you set a **goal**, whether it's to start exercising or learn how to cook, your brain kicks dopamine into gear the moment you anticipate that goal. Pretty cool, right? That's because your brain loves **rewards**. And when you outline what you want to achieve, it's like telling your brain, "Hey, good stuff is coming!" That whole process starts getting dopamine flowing, and as a result, you feel more motivated to chase that goal.

Now, let's dive a little deeper. Picture this: you've just decided you're going to finish reading an entire novel this month. At first, it's all thrill and excitement—the mere thought of completing it triggers your dopamine response. This **anticipation** is everything. Your brain gets hyped about the journey you're about to embark on, much like how a kid feels walking into a candy store. The image of flipping that last page is your brain's dangling carrot, teasing you with a pay-off that's worth the effort. And every small step you take towards reaching that goal—like finishing a chapter here and there—gives your dopamine levels a little bump, making you eager to keep going.

But there's more to it than just setting the goal. Simply having the goal sitting there on your to-do list isn't enough. The real magic lies in noticing **progress**. When you're halfway through that novel or an hour deep into learning how to perfect your lasagna recipe, you're feeding your brain with little hits of dopamine each time you knock a task off or make some actual progress. And that's where the dopamine-motivation cycle really ramps up. You do something small, get a tiny reward, and guess what? You're suddenly re-energized, ready to take on the next part of the goal. This creates a positive feedback loop. It's like lighting a spark, and then watching it smolder with every bit of progress until, boom, a full-on fire gets going. It's that urge to go the extra mile because you're seeing results that keeps feeding the process.

And this brings us to structuring your goals in a way that maximizes dopamine—let's call this a Dopamine-Optimized Goal Structure. To get the most out of this brain-driven **motivation**, you've got to think a bit differently about how you set those goals. Start by making them super clear and, more importantly, tiny. I mean really small. Each mini-goal needs to be specific but something you can nail within a short time. Mastering that short, sharp task means you instantly get a little dopamine kick. For instance, instead of saying you want to lose 20 pounds—try celebrating when you lose 5 or even 2. These incremental goals should be packed with tangible results, something you can measure or see. Having checkpoints like that makes sure you're constantly feeding the brain its happy juice.

And don't forget to throw in a little **reward** system. Even just marking off tasks on a list can be like handing yourself a gold star—totally dopamine-worthy! The structure revolves around defining clear steps, tracking progress with those celebrations in-between, and keeping the big goals in view, but never losing focus on those dopamine-hitting wins along the way. Soon, that pathway to your final goal isn't only possible; it's pretty darn addictive.

Breaking Down Large Goals for Consistent Dopamine Boosts

When you're staring at a really **big goal** - you know, like getting your health where you want it or finishing a long project - it's easy to feel overwhelmed. The target feels so far off; it's like trying to climb a never-ending mountain. Every time you take a step, the peak doesn't seem any closer. That's where you might get stuck while trying to be productive. But there's actually a neat trick that takes that giant avalanche of a goal and smooths it out into something more, well, actionable. It's all about making those huge, intimidating goals look more approachable by chipping them into smaller pieces that you can handle day by day.

Instead of aiming straight for the top, cut it up into bits that feel way more doable. Ask yourself a simple question: What's the tiniest action you can take that starts you on that journey? Do it. Then do another one tomorrow. You start small and watch the **progress** roll in as ticking off each item on your list creates a sense of accomplishment. Honestly, tricking your own brain into feeling like you're winning even though you have this monster of a goal ahead is the name of the game. Every time you accomplish one of those smaller tasks, no matter how small it is, you're rewarded with a little spike of **dopamine**—a win-dose—and it's the crack you need for sustained **motivation**.

Imagine you're running a marathon but you break it into tiny miles. If at each mile, you tell yourself, "Okay, as long as I make it here..." before you know it, you'll get all the way across. Instead of waiting 'til you hit the finish line to let that dopamine kick in, you're getting a bit of that lovely neurotransmitter with every step forward. **Momentum** suddenly drives itself; it fuels up on its way there, which makes the initially nearly impossible journey seem surprisingly manageable.

This all nicely shifts into the real meat here—Dopamine Milestone Mapping. That sounds techy or something, right? It's actually a super clever way to keep giving yourself dopamine treats while getting closer to your major goals. Basically, you map out a series of mini-goals, or **milestones**, each offering something to look forward to. These are concrete tasks you can accomplish and they fit together like steps on a ladder leading up to your ultimate goal. Nothing too complex is happening here—just more small wins you feed on to keep that positivity up and steady.

So, let's say you're looking to write a whole **book**—a big task by any standard. Don't fool yourself into thinking you're going to wake up in the next month and just have it done. But how about writing one chapter a week? How about setting your first milestone at just drafting the outline? You get there, that's a win already which fuels your motivation to get to the next milestone—maybe doing the research. Slice through that bad-boy of a task into edible chunks, and every chunk you finish offers you a bit of that dopamine reward.

What's happening here is you're fooling your brain into thinking "I'm progressing!" when, technically, this long process would have been hard to push through if that finish line seemed just terribly out of reach. Breaking down this goal is like stacking bricks that keep giving you a tiny shot of **motivation** every time one is laid. Before you know it, your goal isn't a mountain anymore. It's a staircase.

Acknowledging Small Wins to Maintain Motivation

Celebrating small victories might sound like an afterthought, but it's one of those little habits that can make a **big difference** in keeping your motivation rolling. It's like a nudge, reminding your brain that you're moving in the right direction—even when you're not where you want to be just yet. The thing is, every time you give yourself a little pat on the back, your brain releases that hit of dopamine, which feels good and keeps you going. Think of it like a **snowball effect**. Once you get those dopamine-driven actions going, they just kind of build on themselves, each win propelling you to tackle the next challenge. It's that simple but effective cycle of "do something, feel good, do more." Who doesn't want to keep that cycle alive?

But here's the thing—you've gotta make these celebrations meaningful if they're going to pack the punch you're looking for. It's not just about rewarding yourself for the sake of it—it's about figuring out what actually matters to you. Because let's be real, handing yourself a meaningless reward won't have the same **impact** as something that really speaks to your values or aligns with your bigger goals. Got a goal you're pumped about? Pair that with a reward that fits. If your big dream is running a marathon, maybe treat yourself to a new running playlist after hitting a milestone, rather than something that doesn't connect with your objectives. The trick is making sure that the rewards you choose match up with the **progress** you're trying to make. That way, you don't just feel good in the moment—you keep that forward momentum.

So how do you set up this whole reward system thing in a way that's both effective and, well, fun? Enter the "Dopamine-Friendly Reward System." An important part of making any goal-setting process work is knowing when and how to give yourself some credit—and how to use that credit wisely. It's all about setting up cool **incentives** that don't just fit your goals but also keep you excited paired with the dopamine rush they bring. Start by breaking down your big goal into smaller, digestible chunks. Each time you complete one, take a second to acknowledge it. That's step one— just recognizing, genuinely, that you accomplished something.

At the same time, pick a reward system that makes sense for you. Maybe collecting points that lead up to a larger, more meaningful treat. Or perhaps a small indulgence for each milestone—within reason, of course—might be more your style. It's kind of like flipping an internal switch, sending a message to your brain: "Hey, you're on the right track, keep this up!" Just make sure your rewards don't derail you from your main goal. The reward should enhance your **motivation**, not leave you scrambling to catch up again. Balance is key—snagging a reward while still keeping the bigger picture in view. It's all about keeping your head in the game without losing sight of the end zone.

So, all in all, it's about **patience**, persistence, and giving yourself credit where it's due. When you focus on recognizing those wins, get clever about rewarding yourself, and have a system in place that feels good, you're setting yourself up for a chain reaction of motivation. Each little success pulls you—little by little—closer to where you want to be. And in that, my friend, you'll find the steady burn of real, lasting **motivation**.

Overcoming Setbacks without Dopamine Crashes

You know that sweet **high** you get when you tick a goal off your list, right? It's that rush of **accomplishment** making you feel like you can conquer anything. But what about those times when things don't go so smoothly? When setbacks hit like a ton of bricks, it's easy for your brain to crash – dragging your **dopamine** levels along with it. That's a rough spot. And keeping your **motivation** alive during these moments... well, that takes some work, doesn't it?

One way to keep that drive burning bright, even when times are tough, is to change how you look at setbacks. You might view failures as massive roadblocks, unable to move past them. They seem impossible to overcome. But here's what's really key – try seeing them as learning moments instead. Think about what didn't work or what you could do differently next time. It's about not letting yourself spiral down. You keep things steady that way. When you shift your focus like this, setbacks start to look less like defeats and more like opportunities. Sure, it sounds easier said than done, but with practice, it gets manageable.

So, how do you actually do it? Well, when you hit a snag, pause and take a deep breath. Don't go straight to self-blame or **frustration**. Start by asking yourself a simple question: "What can I learn from this?" This little shift in thought can make sure your dopamine levels don't take a wild nosedive. Stay curious. Treat each setback like a puzzle – something to figure out, not something to fear. And when you crack that puzzle, that's when real **growth** happens.

Once you've got this mindset in check, the next step is having a "Stay Motivated Plan." Planning out how you'll tackle setbacks beforehand means you'll be ready for them. And by doing that, you basically bulletproof your drive.

A good "Stay Motivated Plan" should have these elements:

• Revisit Your "Why": Remind yourself of the reasons you started working toward your goal in the first place. What were you excited about in the beginning? Reconnecting with that original passion can reignite the flame and keep you moving forward.

• Set Mini-Goals: Big goals are overwhelming. Break them down into bite-sized steps instead. Each small victory gives you that little dopamine hit without weighing you down. And this keeps momentum going.

• Surround Yourself with Positivity: Whether it's a close friend, a favorite book, or a simple playlist, keep things around you that lift your spirits. It's tough to stay motivated when you're surrounded by doom and gloom, after all.

• Practice Gratitude: Sometimes a setback can really shake you. Take a moment, write down a few things you're thankful for – even on bad days. These little reminders work wonders in keeping your optimism in check.

Moving from one point to another like this, the laziness that blows in from setbacks gets shut out fast. Those small wins pile up, keeping your head above water.

Lastly, let's recognize that setbacks aren't just temporary roadblocks. They hold precious lessons for when you start heading towards your next venture. And with the right frame of mind, they won't pull you into a dopamine crash, but rather, have the potential (if you allow) to boost your **growth** much more than any initial success. Yes, setbacks stink. But they're incredible teachers when you let them be.

So, remember – **success** isn't just about constantly winning; it's about battling through those losses, keeping your mood up, and never letting the lows paralyze your high.

Practical Exercise: Creating a Dopamine-Friendly Goal System

Setting the right **goals** can feel like trying to build a puzzle without seeing the final picture. The pieces are everywhere, and it's easy to get caught up in tasks that aren't getting you closer to what truly matters. That's where a solid **plan** helps—especially one that plays nice with the way your brain wants to motivate you. Today, we're talking about creating a system that leverages your dopamine levels for maximum payout.

So, let's start by figuring out what really matters to you. Long-term goals that actually mean something—those are the ones that stick. They're the ones that align with your values, giving you a sense of **purpose** and direction. Take a little time to think about your life right now. What are the things that genuinely bring you fulfillment, things you'd be proud to have said you achieved? These aren't those fleeting desires fueled by envy or boredom, but the anchors that guide your life. The big picture stuff.

Maybe you're into helping others—you'd value a career that leaves a social impact. Or maybe you cherish freedom and would be happier crafting a lifestyle that lets you work and play on your own terms. This is step one because without a grounded sense of what you actually care about, all the planning in the world won't keep you motivated.

Moving on—you don't have to climb the whole mountain at once. Every mountain has a series of small steps that help you steadily make your way to the summit. Once your long-term goals are clear, it's time to chop them into bite-sized pieces. Stuff that you can see, measure, and feel good about completing. Say, if the long-term goal is a health thing, like better **fitness**, then smaller goals might be weekly steps like prepping meals or committing to jog a certain distance. Smaller goals make it manageable.

Each little win triggers a dopamine release, a little "atta boy!" from your brain that says, "Nice, keep it up." And since we're aiming to work with your brain chemistry here, those small victories are critical for keeping you pumped about continuing your progress.

Alright, so everything's broken down. What's next? It's time to set clear **deadlines** for each of these smaller goals. Assigning a timeframe to these tasks makes them real and pushes you to actually get them done, rather than letting things drift. Plus, there's something genuinely motivating about seeing a measurable drop in days to achieve something, and that little "oh wow, only three days left" moment is dopamine gold waiting to happen. Just don't cram too many goals into tight spaces—allow yourself some breathing room to succeed without unnecessary pressure.

To really lock everything in place, take those steps from your long-term map to success and toss them up on something visual. Could be a calendar, a simple chart—you don't need to overcomplicate it. Just something that you can check day-to-day, something that reminds you of where you're headed, showing you the steps you've already stomped on. It kinda solidifies the whole thing, seeing your movie take shape visually. It also teases future milestones to target, keeping the excitement burning.

But visualizing isn't enough if you don't measure how you're doing! Set up a way to keep **track** of progress. This can be as easy as checking off a list. Remember those weight trackers where you color in blocks? That principle, applied to any goal, taps into how much humans love seeing proof of effort—what you've built already, concrete steps you've nailed. It brings a sense of satisfaction and keeps the momentum rolling. But don't beat yourself up if the progress is slow or if you decide to tweak the drafts. It's all part of the game.

At the end, make it feel **rewarding**. Hitting milestones deserves a treat—a little something that's meaningful to you, but nothing excessive. Maybe every time you tick off a goal, there's a weekend getaway waiting for you, or something as simple as indulging in your favorite activity. The reward becomes another tool to boost those dopamine levels, reinforcing your hard work and pushing you to keep grinding.

Now, don't go treating this like it's set in stone. Sit down every now and then, look back, reflect, and ask yourself if this system still makes sense. Goals change. Life shifts. Keep it fluid. Timely check-ins help ensure that progress feels good, not forced. It's these little tweaks that ensure goals aren't dragging you but instead pulling you forward naturally, with your brain happily being a cooperative companion on this journey to something that is genuinely **meaningful** to you.

In Conclusion

This chapter sheds light on the tight-knit relationship between **goal-setting** and dopamine—a crucial brain chemical that fuels your **motivation**. Getting a handle on how your goals impact dopamine can help you stay pumped and step up your game when it comes to achieving what you set out to do. By breaking down big goals into bite-sized chunks, giving yourself a pat on the back for your wins, and keeping threats to your drive in check, you're building a solid system that keeps you moving forward.

You've seen how setting and nailing goals triggers dopamine in your brain, and how **progress** and anticipation are key players in keeping your fire burning over the long haul. You've learned the value of chopping up large goals into smaller, easy-to-reach milestones that give you a steady dopamine boost. You've also discovered the impact of **celebrating** even the small victories to keep your engine running, and picked up strategies to bounce back from setbacks without tanking your dopamine levels.

This chapter has armed you with tools to make **goal-setting** a process that supercharges your motivation. Try putting these techniques into action, take baby steps forward, and cherish each **accomplishment**. Over time, you'll find yourself not only smashing your goals more effectively but also enjoying the ride. **Bright futures** are built on consistent efforts, and every step forward counts!

So, roll up your sleeves and get cracking. Your **future self** will thank you for the **dopamine-fueled journey** you're about to embark on!

Chapter 12: Creativity and Dopamine Flow

Ever wondered why those moments of **creativity** always leave you buzzing with energy? As I sat with my notebook one morning, lost in a wave of fresh ideas, I couldn't help but think... What if there's more to it than just inspiration striking? You see, I believe creativity doesn't only change the way you think; it floods your **brain** with something even more powerful—**dopamine**. And you, too, have access to this incredible boost whenever you engage in creative activities—whether it's painting, writing, or solving puzzles.

In this chapter, we're going to dive into the intricate dance between your brain's **creativity** and dopamine levels. By the end, you'll look at everyday **problem-solving** and playful activities in a completely different light. Ready to figure out how to make creativity a daily **habit** that'll keep your **mood** in check? Stick around... there's a lot more to uncover.

You'll discover how tapping into your creative side can be a game-changer for your overall well-being. It's not just about producing art or coming up with innovative ideas; it's about giving your **brain** that sweet dopamine rush that keeps you feeling energized and motivated. So, whether you're a seasoned artist or someone who thinks they don't have a creative bone in their body, this chapter's got something for you. Get ready to unlock the power of your creative mind and harness the feel-good vibes that come with it.

The Connection Between Creativity and Dopamine

Ever tried to come up with a quick solution to a problem and just felt stuck? Like your brain had zero input to offer? That's likely because one of your brain's key players—dopamine—wasn't fully on board. When it comes to creative thinking and solving problems, dopamine has quite the reputation. It's like the **superhero** behind your best ideas, lending you that magical spark you didn't even know you had.

You know that feeling when you've just cracked a difficult problem or stumbled upon a fantastic idea? Well, that little thrill you get—that's dopamine doing its thing. It's like it opens up all the doors in your brain, letting fresh air in and helping you connect dots that maybe weren't even on the same page before. And when those doors are wide open, creativity doesn't just come—it's unleashed. You might find yourself looking at things from different angles or inventing solutions that never crossed your mind before.

Now, when dopamine levels are low, that flow? Not so great. Think of it as struggling to squeeze toothpaste from an almost-empty tube—super frustrating, right? You still have ideas, but they aren't easy to pull out. In fact, they might even seem stuffy or old. But here's where dopamine is just pure **brilliance**. When it's up, you can start piecing things together—recycling some old ideas, sure—but adding something completely new to the mix. It pulls all the cool bits and bobs from your brain, the stuff that, alone, doesn't seem much at first glance. Together? They make something pretty special.

Okay, so imagine you're trying to spice up an old recipe. You've got your usual ingredients, a bit more digging around the kitchen, and boom! You pull out some unexpected items you hadn't actually planned on using... but hey, why not? That's sort of how dopamine helps you think outside the box. It encourages you to "mix it up," if you will, pushing you to try out combinations your comfortable self might shy away from. Without those punches of extra dopamine here and there, the **magic** of discovery isn't quite the same. Sure, maybe the end result won't always be a winner, but you can bet something valuable will come out of it next time.

Now, you might wonder, is creativity just a matter of tweaking how much dopamine we can pump into our system? Well, it's like crafting the right dish—ingredients matter, but just stirring and boiling isn't automatically gonna get you gourmet. You see, creativity doesn't just depend on dopamine; it's how those bursts are shipped around and land in the right spots. Some places in your brain react stronger to dopamine's knock, answering eagerly. These regions are fantastic at seeing new details others miss, more interested in the bigger imaginative picture, so to speak. Their savvy lies in connecting the familiar but finding new processes locked away somewhere quieter.

And to weave this all together? It helps to picture a focus point—a Creativity-Dopamine Synergy Map. (Sorry, but semi-scientific sounding technospeak will pop up in this book, especially heading toward the back chapters). If there's a direct line between bursts of dopamine and bursts of creativity bringing ideas to life—it might look like this: dopamine triggers brain parts that shred old ideas and pop new, shiny ones in. Each section then sends a message back to connect creativity like levels on a lookout tower. One idea sparks **interest**, another joins the conversation, then adds colors, switches gears, and finally unveils a fresh **perspective**—born right out of nowhere when the mood was just right. So yeah, creativity and dopamine? Inseparable pals driving some of your best **sparks**.

Engaging in Creative Activities for Dopamine Balance

Sometimes, what's missing in your life is a splash of **creativity**—the kind that naturally puts you in a good mood. You know that little rush you feel when you finish drawing something cool or finally write that poem you've been thinking about? That's **dopamine** in action. Engaging in creative activities releases this feel-good chemical in your brain, which can be a healthy way to manage how you feel without reaching for unhealthy habits.

If you're looking for ways to get that **boost** without relying on your social media accounts or junk food, creativity is your best bet. You don't have to be a painter, a poet, or even have experience in creative fields to activate this. Everyone can tap into it, no matter what floats their boat. Whether you're picking up an old hobby or trying something completely different, the key is to have fun with it.

Even the little things like doodling or playing with colors in adult coloring books can do wonders for your **mood**. Don't think big pressure—think small wins. Perhaps you'll find joy in making handmade birthday cards or trying your hand at a new recipe just for the heck of it.

But how does being creative regularly balance things out? Well, think of it like a scorecard you're keeping with your brain. The more you engage in creative activities, the less likely you are to feel low or out of sorts. Dopamine is released in small, steady bursts that keep you from hitting those extremes, whether high or low—like stepping on a seesaw, but with mental control. Come up with a list of enjoyable activities that make you feel like, "Wow, I've got this," and sprinkle them throughout your weeks. The trick? Keep them varied and fresh. Different creative avenues lead to different bursts of dopamine, each giving your brain a teachable moment in its own way. No room for boredom here.

So, about that list? I've got a bunch of ideas that'll help you tap into **creativity** without overcomplicating stuff. I like to think of it as a "Dopamine-Boosting Creative Activity Menu." Curious? Here, let me lay it out for you:

• Painting/Drawing: Doodling, grabbing paint, or even getting into digital art can awaken colors in your mind, which triggers dopamine while improving concentration.

• Journaling/Free Writing: Let words flow—no structure needed. Pour out your thoughts, and who knows? You might surprise yourself with some deep realization from those spontaneous scribbles.

• Cooking/Baking: Don your apron and try out that weird combo recipe from Pinterest. Combining ingredients in new ways does wonders for your senses, rewarding your brain with dopamine bursts as flavors meld.

• Knitting or Crochet: Might seem like your grandma's thing, but there's something so calming yet satisfying about creating a scarf, blanket, or anything that adds a pop of color.

• DIY Crafts: From building birdhouses to assembling photo frames, crafting regular little projects lets you add your personal touch—because you literally create something out of nothing.

• Music: Try composing, remixing, or learning an **instrument**. Your brain lights up in multiple ways when you're involved in producing something musical, even if it's just strumming a few chords on an acoustic guitar.

• Photography: Get outdoors or use stuff around the house. Capturing moments or staging scenes stimulates not only your sight but your brain's entire reward system.

Changing things up by dabbling in various creative outlets keeps those dopamine vibes flowing. Keep the **momentum** going, and notice how these fun endeavors accumulate, keeping your mood and mind strong.

It's this combination of routine and variety that does the trick. On some days, your focus could be organizing pictures—while on others, it might be writing short poems about your day. Little efforts make a big difference, and by regularly engaging in these activities, you'll start to see less reliance on external thrills and more excitement over your creativity. Creativity not only stabilizes your mood but also gives life meaning during those inevitable stints of gray days when motivation runs dim. That sense of **achievement** you'll feel—well, I've already mentioned the dopamine rewards, but there's also this quiet sense that life's good because you're doing something that means something to you.

So, jot down your list, start easy, and just have fun. Trust me, your dopamine levels are loving it already.

Problem-Solving as a Dopamine Booster

You know that **rush** you get when you crack a tough nut? That's your brain's way of giving you a high-five with a sweet dose of dopamine. Tackling complex problems isn't just about finding solutions; it's like feeding your **brain** a tasty treat. Seriously, your gray matter gets a kick out of a good puzzle.

When you're faced with a multi-layered challenge, your brain goes into overdrive—connecting dots, testing theories, and figuring stuff out. In return, it showers you with dopamine, the stuff that makes you feel like a million bucks. The **problems** don't have to be earth-shattering; it could be crafting the perfect email, nailing a Sudoku, or mapping out the ultimate road trip. As long as it gets your **gears** turning, you're in for that sweet dopamine kick.

Here's where it gets juicy: the tougher the problem, the bigger the **reward**. Your brain loves piecing together a mental jigsaw puzzle. It's playing the long game; that final "eureka!" moment unleashes a flood of feel-good chemicals. This doesn't just make problem-solving satisfying; it **motivates** you to take on even bigger challenges next time. You're literally rewiring your brain to crave these dopamine hits when you **think** through a problem.

But wait, there's more! Tackling intellectual challenges is like hitting the gym for your brain—keeping it sharp and fit. This mental workout actually beefs up the connections in your noggin. Picture it like a trail in the woods; the more you hike it, the clearer it becomes. The more you flex those problem-solving muscles, the easier it gets for your brain to tackle future **challenges**.

It's a win-win: you solve a problem and buff up your brain in the process. This doesn't just keep you mentally sharp; it gives your overall mood a serious boost. The intellectual satisfaction paired with that dopamine surge works wonders for your spirits. Think of it as training your brain the same way you'd keep your body in shape—you're investing in your mental health while getting hooked on tackling tough tasks.

Now, imagine if you could get all these perks with a roadmap to guide you. That's where the "Dopamine-Driven Problem-Solving Framework" comes in—yeah, it's a mouthful, but stick with me. It's a flexible structure to help you break problems into bite-sized chunks. Feel free to tweak it to suit your style. The gist? You'll brainstorm, organize your ideas, test them out, and reflect on what works.

It's like a mini-adventure for your brain, with dopamine boosts along the way. Each step in the framework gives you a little pat on the back, nudging you towards the solution. Start by pinpointing what makes the problem tricky. Then, let your mind wander and explore possible solutions without judgment. This free-wheeling brainstorming taps into your creative juices, giving your dopamine another chance to flow. Organize your thoughts, test them out, and see how they stack up. Each small win keeps those dopamine levels humming and keeps you pumped throughout the process.

So, in a nutshell, solving problems isn't just about finding answers. It's about nourishing your brain with the rewards it craves—dopamine, motivation, and a healthier mind. Plus, you get that sweet satisfaction of watching something complex unfold before your eyes. Why wait? Go tackle that next problem like a boss.

The Role of Play in Dopamine Regulation

When was the last time you did something just for the **fun** of it? Not because it had to be done or there was a reward waiting for you at the end, but simply to enjoy yourself? Doing fun stuff isn't just for kids – it's actually powerful when it comes to tickling your brain's **dopamine** center. That burst of happiness or that feeling of excitement when you're having a blast? It's not only in your head; it's real, thanks to dopamine.

Whether you're bouncing on a trampoline, doodling in a sketchbook, or trying out a goofy dance move in your living room – these small moments of **play** aren't merely distractions. They're essential in giving your brain that dopamine spike, lifting your mood along the way. The reason is simple: When you engage in something enjoyable, your brain releases dopamine as a sort of "Hey, this is great!" chemical signal. It makes you want to keep enjoying playful activities and leaves you feeling energized afterward.

That's why it's important to sprinkle these playtime moments throughout your week. Over time, packing your days only full of responsibility and structure can wear you down. Your brain constantly (consciously or otherwise) charts dopamine levels to aim for "normal." If you're just grinding day in and day out? That "normal" level might take a hit. You lose **motivation**, maybe start feeling flat or "meh," and that's even before we jump into how people start sliding into bad habits seeking that dopamine lift elsewhere.

Think of play as more than just a guilty pleasure or waste of time. Actually, your brain sees it as super-charged fuel – the stuff that not only helps keep your dopamine levels balanced but also promotes **creativity** and motivation. Remember this: Life isn't just about ticking off to-dos. It's about carving out little slices of joy and spontaneity, sidestepping the grind for just a few minutes here and there.

Okay, so what now? How do you actually fit this into your life without feeling like it's one more thing to check off? This is where the "Adult Play Prescription" comes in handy.

Adult Play Prescription

Here's the play prescription to help blend these dopamine-boosting moments into your daily groove:

• **Micro-Breaks** — Take out five minutes twice a day where you mess around with nothing other than play. This can be having a dance-off with yourself in front of the mirror or competing with the clock to stack as many random items on your desk as possible.

• **Scheduled Playtime** — Designate specific no-excuse-allowed play slots in your week. Like Sunday afternoons— even if it's baking crazy shaped cookies or building a chair fort, make it mandatory fun.

• **Playful Hobbies** — Incorporate a hobby in your daily routine that you do just 'cause it's fun—gardening (without caring about perfection), collecting random bizarre trinkets, whatever teases out your inner curious child.

Staying connected to playfulness brings that much-needed zest back into your life balance sheet. It won't feel frivolous once you notice the lift in **mood** and motivation sliding through your days. Just don't wrap this all up in shoulds—play because it nurtures that vital thrill and freshness, reminding you, no matter your age, that skipping the daily grind is a-okay for those **serotonin** factories in your head.

Practical Exercise: Integrating Creativity into Daily Life

Time to **level** with yourself. What's up with your current creative activities? Are they **flowing** the way you'd like them to, or is there a bit of a clog in the pipe? The goal here is to see where creativity already fits into your life. Maybe you paint when you're stressed, or you write in a journal before bed—whatever it is, it's part of you. But... could you do more? Probably. Most of us sideline creativity after a while, especially when life ramps up the tempo with to-do lists and responsibilities.

Start by taking a good look at where your **creativity** fits at the moment. Where does it show up? And more importantly, where's it missing? Are there gaps in your everyday where you could sneak in a bit more creativity? It could be that ten-minute window every morning while you wait for the coffee to brew. That's a good spot to insert a sketch or a haiku. By recognizing these gaps, you'll begin to see opportunities that've always been there—they just needed a bit of dusting off.

Once you know where creativity is, and where it's lacking, figure out what you'd like to add to your **routine**. And that brings us to the next step: time to dip your toe into the waters of something completely new. Every week, try out a different creative activity— something outside your norm. It doesn't have to be anything grandiose; it could be as simple as doodling in the margins or trying your hand at making clay figures. The point is to shake things up and step out of your usual comfort zone.

Some of these creative jaunts might click with you while others might be more suited for the back burner—or even the frozen tundra of 'never again.' But that's fine. Each time you try something new, you open another valve to pump more dopamine into your life. It's always interesting to see which new activity sticks.

Alright, you've identified the gaps, explored something new each week. Now it's important to carve out **time** specifically for these creative endeavors. If we're being honest, whatever isn't scheduled has a way of sliding into Neverland. So, when exactly are you making time to be creative? Morning, before the day's got its claws in you? Maybe the hour before bed when things have finally quieted down? The when doesn't matter as much as making sure it's there—and it's protected, like a vault lining your mental wellbeing.

Without a dedicated time slot, creativity tends to be that thing you'll "get to eventually"...only "eventually" never comes. Slot time in. Commit to it like you would an important meeting, because—let's be real—it is. This is your dedicated time to let the brain wander, unravel ideas, and essentially, boost your mood a little.

Now, creating space in your day is one thing, but creating **space** in your environment's another ballgame—and just as crucial. This could be as simple as finding a cozy nook in your living room corner that's punctuated with whatever tools you use, whether that's a bunch of pencils, a slew of notebooks, or just a comfy floor cushion where daydreaming flows like a river.

Don't underestimate the power of having a dedicated creativity corner. Seriously, having space for all your creative projects nudges you every time you pass by, subtly convincing you to sit down and work on something, even if it's just for five minutes. Piece by piece, that dedicated nook becomes almost like a mini-altar where creative energy hangs tight, always in the air.

You've got the hang of it now. But **ideas** are a lot like slippery fish, they get away from you if you don't net them right when you have them. So what's your fishnet, huh? Your phone's notes app? A sketchpad or some stray napkins? It's crucial to keep something handy for jotting down ideas as they come to you throughout the day. Make capturing these ideas a habit. They might flash across your brain while you're in line for coffee or on that boring conference call—grab them before they swim away.

This could involve a bit of daily discipline, corralling those thoughts into an easy-to-reach place where you can come back to them later with a clearer mind. Do this, and you'll find creative projects folding together with a lot less effort.

And then, there's pushing yourself a little farther than feels comfortable. Doesn't sound like fun, does it? But trust me, it's worth it because that's where the **growth** is. Set up "creative challenges" to nudge your boundaries. Nothing extreme, but enough to stretch you beyond just what's easy. Maybe it's committing to sketching 30 portraits in 30 days, or maybe it's filming a 1-minute clip of something every day for a month—whatever heightens the stakes just a touch. Guess what else ramps up? That good ol' dopamine rush when you meet the challenge.

So, look back. Reflect on how these steps have added more zest to your days, how your mood has swayed, and how **motivation** seems to roll easier. Creativity isn't just something extra—it's the oil that smoothens the gears of your mind. When you engage in creative activities, you're brightening your mood, sharpening your motivation, and adding more fun to everything.

Spending more time being creative might even open up parts of yourself you didn't know were closed off before. Keep at it, observe the changes, and see how much more vivid everything—your mood, your energy—gets with a little dose of creativity every day.

In Conclusion

This chapter sheds light on the **powerful** connection between **creativity** and **dopamine**, showing how diving into imaginative activities can boost your mood and sharpen your mind. By triggering dopamine through creative pursuits, you can spark **innovative** problem-solving, balance your emotions, and give your cognitive well-being a serious upgrade. When you explore new avenues for creative expression, you're paving the way to better **brain** health, fighting off stress, and setting yourself up for long-term happiness.

You've seen how creativity and dopamine release go hand in hand, and how playful, unstructured activities can give you a dopamine kick. You've learned that creative exercises can work wonders for your brain's well-being, and that tackling problems head-on stimulates dopamine flow. Plus, you've got some practical tips on how to make **creativity** a regular part of your life to keep those dopamine levels humming.

By putting these ideas into action, you can start weaving creativity into your daily grind, building a healthier mindset and adding a spark to your everyday life. Keep exploring those **hobbies**, seek out **intellectual** challenges, and don't forget to play around— sometimes, the most joyful moments come from letting your **imagination** run wild. So go ahead, unleash your creative side and watch your world light up!

Chapter 13: Sustaining Long-Term Dopamine Balance

Ever wondered why some days feel so **sluggish** while others have that effortless **flow**? I sure have. You know, maintaining that "just right" feeling isn't some mystical art—it's actually pretty achievable. In this chapter, we'll focus on how to keep your mind and body cruising towards a **dopamine** state that lights you up, no matter what's happening around you.

I'll take you through how to form easy **habits** that don't just work today but stick with you as life shifts. Maybe you've hit a wall recently and felt like nothing's budging—that's okay! Together, we'll explore practical ways to push past that. What's more, we'll sprinkle in a bit of **self-compassion** because beating yourself up won't help you in the long run.

You'll learn how to design a dopamine **balance** that feels right to you. It's not about following a one-size-fits-all approach; it's about finding what works for your unique **lifestyle**. We'll dive into strategies that help you maintain that sweet spot of motivation and contentment, even when life throws you curveballs.

Remember, it's all about creating a sustainable approach to managing your **energy** levels. You'll discover how to ride the waves of your natural ups and downs, making the most of your high-energy days and navigating through the low ones with grace.

Ready to embark on this journey towards a more balanced, energized you? Let's dive in and unlock the secrets to sustaining long-term dopamine balance!

Establishing Healthy Habits for Consistent Dopamine Levels

You get it, right? Keeping your dopamine levels steady isn't just like flipping a switch. You can't just spike it and hope to stay balanced over time. It's a long-term game, almost like maintaining a garden where you're constantly watering, weeding, and giving some TLC to keep everything **blooming** nicely. Getting casual spikes in dopamine with things like sugar or social media might feel good for a moment, but they don't last. Instead, those quick fixes can set you on a rollercoaster of highs and lows. Trust me, it doesn't bode well for long-term happiness.

So, enter the holy grail—**routines**. Yeah, the word might sound a bit boring, but routines are way more important than any short-lived dopamine kick. See, your brain loves predictability. When you follow consistent routines that you actually enjoy, your brain learns to anticipate and prepare for the joyful reward. It might be subtle, but over time, that pleasurable anticipation helps keep your dopamine levels more balanced and steady. It's like training a dog but subtler. If you understand this and act on it, you'll notice day-to-day stuff becomes less of a drag. Because your brain will start automatically rewarding you for completing even the simplest tasks.

Once you realize that habits can help embed balance, you'll maybe wonder how to start building such a lifestyle. It's not as hard as it seems, but you've got to focus on adding natural dopamine enhancers into your daily life in a genuine way. A lot of folks look toward things like **exercise**. Ever heard of the runner's high? Exercise isn't just for fitness; it's one of the best ways to naturally keep your dopamine flowing consistently. And we're not talking marathons here—just a brisk walk could do the trick. Over time, you'll likely notice that regular physical activity increases your daily dopamine fuel. Even better, low-impact exercises like yoga or stretching maintain your dopamine without pushing your body or brain into overdrive.

And it's not just about moving your body though—what you fuel it with is crucial, too. Eating good **food**, packed with nutrients, has more impact on your mood than folks tend to appreciate. You've got stuff like leafy greens, omega-3 rich foods, nuts, and seeds—they're all dopamine-friendly. Eating "clean" isn't just for Instagram influencers. It really can make a distinction between dragging your heels through the day and having natural energy that doesn't send your mood crashing two hours later. Call it conscious eating if that helps make it sound better, but when you fuel your body right, your dopamine levels thank you for it.

Okay, so we've talked about moving and fueling, yet there's one more piece—something I like to call the Dopamine-Balancing Daily **Ritual**. It's simple but mindfully set up to keep everything flowing steady.

In the morning, get yourself some natural **light**; even just 15 minutes outside sets your body clock and helps regulate dopamine production for the day. Move around, maybe do light exercise or just stretch out. After that, dive into a small task that makes you feel accomplished—it could be as simple as making your bed. Midday, be sure to eat a balanced meal; we're talking protein mixed with complex carbs—whole foods that leave no room for greasy distractions. Hydrate. Then, focus on having at least one mindful moment. Whether through meditation, journaling, or just stepping away from a screen. Winding down the day should involve minimizing exposure to **stimulants**. That means lowered lights, deep breathing, or maybe winding down with some familiar TV show requiring minimal mental effort—the key thing here is relaxation. This daily outline helps provide structure but also flexibility—something your brain loves—and most of all, keeps that dopamine on a level plane.

So, while hopping onto the trendiest apps or high-sugar habits might look inviting, creating simple, natural routines actually sustains long-term **happiness**. It's slow and steady, but hey—just like in the story of the tortoise and the hare, it's often the more sustainable option that wins.

Adjusting Strategies as Life Changes

Life is like riding waves. Sometimes you're **cruising** along smoothly, and other times you're getting tossed around like nobody's business. The same thing happens with your **dopamine** levels—one-size-fits-all just doesn't work forever. What used to fill you with energy might make you yawn a year from now. You have to adjust your **strategies** if your favorite techniques aren't delivering that brain buzz anymore.

Maybe when you were younger, smashing that gym session every morning **pumped** you up for the whole day. But now? Maybe not so much. There's a trick to knowing when it's time to change your methods: listen to your brain and how it reacts. Are you getting that old feeling when you cross things off your to-do list? If it's feeling bland or like a chore instead of a thing that's great, maybe your dopamine strategies are past their prime.

Changing life stages means that what worked before might suddenly stop doing the trick. When you notice things like feeling more **fatigued** or getting irritated by activities that used to be fun, that's a clue. The good news? You can tweak things without starting from scratch. Instead of hitting that gym the same way every day, maybe you need to shift gears. Try trading some intense workouts for a tranquil walk or a yoga session now and then.

That leads us perfectly into a key component of this—recognizing when what you're doing isn't **cutting** it anymore and feeling cool with altering your dopamine strategy. Think of it this way: when you're driving and getting all those road signs, you have the option to change your route. You wouldn't just ignore the signs and keep taking the same turns, would you? Just like with anything in life, you've got to adjust your handling when you see certain indicators like boredom, irritability, or even a sense of flatness.

Here's another example. If you absolutely lived for the rush of tackling everything at work early in your career but stopped feeling fulfilled after a while, that's your brain sending you a memo, saying, "Hey, time to switch it up." That rush you craved isn't cutting it anymore, so you've logically got to switch pathways. Try seeking out newer **challenges** or starting to tackle things beyond work that light up your dopamine system. Who knows, maybe it's time for a new hobby or some creative project that snaps you out of the monotony?

Now, let's talk about a plan. I like to think of the "Dopamine Strategy Flexibility Plan" like keeping a toolbox handy. One technique isn't going to fix every leak that crops up over the years, right? So, on those days you wake up feeling off—like your strategies aren't firing the way they used to—check your toolbox and pick out a new tool. Maybe it's something small like switching up your morning routine, adding a bit of **mindfulness** to it. Or you dive into something completely new, enough to reinvigorate that sense of discovery. No matter what, being flexible in how you regulate your dopamine means paying attention to shifts in your life and adapting to them as needed.

You see, with a little practice, you can get really good at knowing when to swap out tools. It's like maintaining balance on a surfboard—small adjustments, lightweight tweaks here and there, but always trying to stay standing. You're not looking to master one-size-fits-all; you're looking to **adapt**.

Overcoming Plateaus in Dopamine Regulation

You know how it feels when you're **working** hard to keep your dopamine levels steady, and it's all going great — until suddenly, it's not? That's a plateau. It hits you harder than you'd expect, shaking up all the **progress** you've fought so hard to make. All those awesome habits that made you feel **motivated**, driven, and on top of the world start feeling like nothing special. It's frustrating as hell. Your **concentration** slips back into old distracting habits, and your mood follows right behind.

Think of it like a treadmill — at some point, your body and brain get too used to the speed, and suddenly, running isn't as much of a **challenge** anymore. It's flat. Unshifted gears. Your system isn't responding the way it used to, no matter how much you push it.

The thing about dopamine is that your body can adapt to balance super quickly — sometimes too quickly. Even your brain wiring gets used to it, leaving you stuck with zero **change** or growth despite all the effort. Without a few tweaks, the motivation you had for so long just fizzles out. It's not working right anymore, so how do you get yourself back on track?

Instead of getting discouraged — and yeah, we're leaving self-pity out of this one — there are some steps you can take to shake things up. You want to recalibrate your efforts and haul yourself over that wall. If it feels like you're chipping away at a mountain that's stopped responding to your hammer, it's time to swap the hammer for a crowbar. Jiggle things around a bit to make real **progress** again.

Start by changing up your dopamine strategy. Habits and routines are great until they're not — until they're just routine. Your brain craves change to stay hooked, motivated, and happy. Dare I say it, you might need to introduce something novel or stimulating into your regular routines. It can be as simple as altering your exercise routine, adding a new skill to learn, or throwing in a reward system that catches you by surprise. New experiences generate fresh **excitement** — the jolt you need to reseed that lustful dopamine fountain. Consider finding joy even from minor new tasks. Find new music. Take new routes to work. Buy the bread you've never picked up before.

All this isn't just whimsy... There's sound reason behind it. The brain responds to novelty, and this customary interruption reboots your dopamine regulation efforts — shakes off the grime gathered during the superstar-stage of habitual routine. Converting those small creative inputs into bigger motivators doesn't just happen immediately either... Sometimes, you have to re-promote your mood playlist after weeks to actually stick on repeat. See it as rewiring — coding delightful updates into the regulations-heavy neural zones of steady dopamine. It's progressive fun, intense exposure repositioned.

Enter the Dopamine Reset Protocol... The key is to step back before proceeding full throttle. Give yourself a couple of days to release the tension building in your efforts and see if it recalibrates. It's like laying flat on a chiropractor's table and allowing everything to sink back into alignment against natural curves. Shift down to slower routines. This cooldown, blended with later-introduced, brand new tasks, helps reboot your system naturally. Not with fresh rounds of relentless tech gadgets or binging on distractions but with control steady enough to adjust troubleshooting gears more evenly.

Forget leaping ahead as before — instead, restart low and slow for full throttle, savoring dopamine-related uplifts carefully reactivated afterward. Even curiosity should have practical input without forcing gum into a grinder needing refuel every moment you turn distracted. Uplifting setbacks replay precisely in your efforts-to-output rediscovery dance. Now, reconnect during lighter resets reimplanting gentler dopamine tips redesigned via deliberate pausing... Intentionally recalibrated, patient revolutions still power-loaded.

Facing a plateau? Dump older instinct or knee-jerk responses behind dopamine disruptions speedily. Instead, focus strength elsewhere. Test different options leading fast signals towards results delayed over resistant reluctance previously paired around efforts overly ordered and ripened. Common bounce-back routines might not surface those soft primes around sloughed aggregators or causal stuck-thought barriers lately pressed against shifts like stoneweights leading deep progress—slow smart reassignment reacting better matured bearings indigent toward reset grounds.

When you're not pushing too fast? Reset alertness some! Cultivating calmer resolve, unleash resurrected realizations more firmly, retrigger pointers prioritized within dopamine and coping fields gradually revisited subject affinities... The reset calls back processed tearaways tightened slowly moderate payload, leaning into neurology sound-swapped pauses dominance renewed.

The Value of Self-Compassion in Maintaining Balance

When things don't go exactly as planned, it's easy to fall into the trap of **beating** yourself up. Maybe you didn't do as well as you wanted on a project, or maybe you skipped a workout that you'd promised yourself you'd stick to. These moments can cause your stress levels to shoot up, yanking your dopamine balance out of whack. Funny how hard you can judge yourself, isn't it? But being kind to yourself during these times... Well, that makes a world of difference.

Self-compassion helps keep your **dopamine** levels steady. When something goes sideways or when you're feeling down, showing a little understanding towards yourself can really help you bounce back faster. Imagine giving yourself the same grace you'd offer a good friend who's having a rough time. Guess what? That same gentle support works wonders on your brain chemistry too. It's like putting a balm on your soul and letting things heal. Stress lowers, and dopamine—the feel-good chemical in your brain—finds a better balance.

So, being kind to yourself means cutting yourself enough slack to stay **motivated** and calm. It also builds resilience. See, it's a lot easier to keep going if you know you're not gonna beat yourself up with mental sticks every time you mess up. When you practice self-compassion, you maintain a steady flow of dopamine, which in turn keeps you feeling more stable and motivated.

But how do you actually get used to being nice to yourself—especially when those self-critical thoughts sneak in so easily? It's one thing to say "be kind to yourself," but making that a **habit** takes a bit more effort.

One neat way to develop a more compassionate inner voice is to start small. Instead of jumping into changing your whole mindset in one go—a mission that sounds exhausting—just focus on silencing that inner critic whenever it starts nagging. When "I'm not good enough" or "I should have done better" thoughts roll in, pause. Stop what you're doing and just notice. You don't have to fight the thought, but you don't need to accept it as the truth either. Just allow yourself a moment to think about what you'd tell a close friend in the same shoes. Would you say, "Wow, you really messed that up"? Not likely. You'd probably reply with something like, "You did your best, and it's okay to try again." Why not try that on for size when dealing with your latest goof?

It ain't easy, especially if you're used to being tough on yourself. But here's a simple exercise—or more like a practice you can get into—called the "Self-Compassion Dopamine Boost Technique." It's all about staying **balanced** when emotions run high, helping you stay positive and on track whenever life gets a little rocky.

This technique starts with a deep breath. Just one, mindful and slow. In—long and deep, then out—nice and easy. After that, go ahead and say to yourself something along the lines of: "It's okay to not have this all figured out now. It's all a bit hard, but it's not the end of the world. I'll do what I can." Simple words, but they change everything. They create space for a shift.

Next, visualize a time when you accomplished something you were proud of. Dwell on it. That tiny hit of dopamine reminding you could be all you need to get back on your feet and build the **courage** to take on the hard stuff again. In those tough times when you feel overwhelmed and your confidence is wavering, this little trick serves as your reset button. It's not about sweeping failures under the rug. Nope. It's about allowing yourself to move on from them, stronger and a bit wiser.

So yeah, self-compassion isn't just fluffy talk or trendy jargon. It's this thread that weaves into every part of your well-being, helping manage **stress** and keeping that dopamine flow in check. It's about giving yourself the same gentleness that you would with anyone else you care about. By doing that, you stabilize both your emotions and motivation, paving the way to sustain long-term balance. Days when things feel off suddenly become a little easier to take on, all because you reminded yourself you're human. Quashing the inner critic and bringing **kindness** into your own life brings way more than peace—it keeps you motivated, helps keep stress at bay, and keeps your dopamine levels humming at just the right frequency.

Practical Exercise: Designing Your Personalized Dopamine Balance Plan

Congratulations on reaching the point where you're ready to **design** your own Dopamine Balance Plan. Before diving in, take a moment to reflect on what you've learned so far. You've covered everything from defining dopamine to practical ways of managing it daily. By now, you understand that dopamine isn't just about quick rewards; it's more complex, playing a huge role in planning, **motivation**, mood regulation, and your ability to experience pleasure.

The first step is identifying your strengths and **challenges**. Maybe you excel at setting up nature-based routines for steady dopamine hits, like morning walks or creative hobbies. But perhaps resisting the urge to devour a whole sleeve of cookies after a rough day is still a work in progress. That's okay—everyone has their struggles. Knowing where you shine and where you falter provides a solid foundation for your plan.

Next, list out the dopamine **strategies** that resonate with you the most. Perhaps meditation leaves you feeling like a chilled-out superhero, or maybe mindful breathing isn't your cup of tea, but connecting with buddies over board games really lights up your day. Jot these down—both the hits and the misses. They'll serve as your playbook.

Setting up a structure to monitor your well-being is key. Don't sweat it; you don't need fancy timers or color-coded spreadsheets (unless that's your jam). Find something you'll stick to—a weekly journaling habit, a smartphone app that tracks your moods, or just a Sunday night check-in with a good cuppa. The goal isn't perfection but consistency in checking in, tweaking what's not working, and reinforcing what is.

While going solo is doable, having an **accountability** partner can level up your plan from "meh" to "this actually works!" This could be a friend with similar goals or someone who knows when to give you a gentle nudge or a high-five. Virtual groups or quick weekly text check-ins—whatever flows naturally for you.

Stay up-to-date with the latest **dopamine** research. Your favorite techniques might evolve, and what seemed far-fetched before could become your go-to move. Regularly dip into new books, articles, or podcasts to keep your methods fresh and effective.

Finally, create your Dopamine Balance Manifesto. It sounds grand, but it's really just your personal guidebook. Combine all your insights—your highs, lows, effective strategies, support system, and future plans—into a concise "Dopamine Code" to guide your daily choices. Include mantras like "Nature in the AM" or "Daily Creative Outlets" as your constants. This will help keep your priorities clear and easy to revisit.

Now, it's time to put pen to paper. Transform what you've learned into something tailored for you. Each step you take is setting you up to make dopamine your ally—gently guiding you through life's inevitable ups and downs with a stable and smile-inducing dopamine balance.

In Conclusion

This chapter has provided **powerful insights** on how to maintain long-term balanced dopamine levels by establishing healthy habits and adapting to different life changes. By sticking to **routines** and promoting a **lifestyle** that supports ongoing dopamine regulation, you can achieve greater mental clarity, focus, and sustained well-being. Remember, it's all about staying **consistent** and being kind to yourself, even when things don't go as planned.

In this chapter, you've seen the importance of daily routines to keep dopamine levels steady, the connection between your lifestyle and natural dopamine regulation, and how to stay flexible and adjust strategies as your life changes. You've also learned about common **challenges** in keeping balanced dopamine levels and how to overcome them, as well as how self-compassion plays a big role in maintaining dopamine balance.

Maintaining long-term dopamine balance isn't just about following a set plan—instead, it's about staying **committed**, making adjustments when necessary, and practicing kindness towards yourself. By applying these **strategies** in your everyday life, you're setting the foundation for better mental health and leading a more balanced life. Keep going, and don't shy away from making changes when needed, because **consistency** leads to lasting balance and happiness.

To Conclude

Throughout this book, the focus has been to help you consciously **shape** the way dopamine functions in your life, allowing you to transition from being controlled by distractions to finding **balance** and fulfillment. By leveraging scientifically-proven techniques, you've learned how to uplift your mood, stay **motivated**, and resist the temptation of negative habits that arise in our modern, hectic world.

You began by grasping how dopamine acts as a chemical messenger in your brain. This **neurotransmitter** influences everything from mood and motivation to decision-making processes. In a world overwhelmed by stimuli, dopamine becomes the culprit in creating habits that leave you endlessly searching for quick bursts of pleasure. Understanding this is the cornerstone for gaining control.

We discussed the dopamine-driven world you live in—full of incessant notifications, social media updates, and instant gratification. You're living in an environment designed to overstimulate the brain, which makes it easy for dopamine to spiral out of control. The need for you to adapt and reset is critical by recognizing how technology impacts your mental health.

Next, the book delved into the balance between pleasure and pain that dopamine regulates. Constant pursuit of short-term pleasures leads to tolerance, pushing long-term balance further out of reach. You learned the importance of restoring this equilibrium and how crucial it is for sustaining joy and satisfaction.

Identifying and recognizing dopamine imbalances formed a practical foundation, where signs of deficiency and excess were highlighted, acknowledging the critical relationship between dopamine and mental health. Self-awareness is paramount for combating any issues.

The **science** of dopamine regulation, rooted in neuroplasticity, gave you insight into the malleability of your brain. Understanding how to adjust dopamine levels through nutrition, **exercise**, sleep, and conscious habits is powerful for fostering long-lasting change.

As we ventured into other techniques—whether it's through diet, spawned by moments of physical activity, consistent sleep patterns, or structured goal setting—we've built essential tools to initiate and maintain practical dopamine management.

Looking forward, when you integrate these learnings into your daily **routine** deliberately, you'll find not just a momentary uplift in mood or motivation, but consistent balance through considered **lifestyle** changes. Imagine reducing anxiety, responding with greater patience, and crafting a life free from the chaos that often feels unmanageable.

If you're eager to deepen your understanding and inspired to take more actionable measures for real change, don't hesitate.

Visit this link to find out more:

https://pxl.to/LoganMind

Join my Review Team!

Thank you for picking up this **book**! Your support means the world to me, and I'd love to hear your thoughts. If you enjoy **reading** and sharing your honest opinions, I'd like to personally invite you to join my Review Team.

As a member, you'll receive a free copy of my upcoming **books** before they hit the shelves, simply in exchange for your honest **feedback**. Your insights are invaluable to me, helping me to produce even better **stories** in the future.

To join the team, you'll need to:

• Click the link below

• Sign up with your email

• Keep an eye out for **notifications** when a new book is releasing

Check out the team at this link:

https://pxl.to/loganmindteam

Help Me!

When you're done reading, if you feel this book has brought you joy, inspiration, or a new perspective, **I'd love to hear from you**! Supporting an independent author like me means supporting a dream, and **your voice matters**.

If you're **satisfied**, please consider leaving an honest review by visiting the link below. If you have **suggestions**, I'm always eager to improve. Feel free to send them to me via the contact information provided at the link.

Every review, no matter how brief, can help others discover and connect with this book. Your **feedback** can leave a lasting impact, not just on me, but on many new readers.

It only takes a few seconds and would mean the **world** to an independent author striving to bring stories to life.

Thank you from the bottom of my heart for your support!

Visit this link to leave a feedback:

https://pxl.to/12-tpod-lm-review

Made in the USA
Las Vegas, NV
01 December 2024

13049382R00095